"Hospitals are enormously complex institutions. This book seeks to de-mystify how they can operate more effectively. Hospital Capacity Management-Insights and Strategies, is an important addition to the literature at a time when many institutions are confronted with a myriad of capacity challenges.

"Dr. Dick and Robert Agness have written a timely book during a time of great stress within the hospital industry. **Hospital Capacity Management: Insights and Strategies**, does a terrific job in describing how hospitals can operate more efficiently and with improved patient care services to meet the capacity challenges of these difficult times.

"The current pandemic has elevated the challenges that hospitals face in meeting the health care demands of the communities that they serve. Dr. Dick and Robert Agness have written a timely book that assists hospital management and consumers alike, in understanding and improving how capacity demands can be met and patient care services improved. This book is an important read for those interested in understanding the complexities of the hospital environment and the steps necessary to meet the challenges of our times."

Steven I. Goldstein, M.H.A.
President & CEO, Strong Memorial Hospital, URMC

"A refreshingly candid and thoughtful look at the state of hospital capacity management in the U.S., and the vital role it plays in driving the healthcare industry's Triple Aim – better care, better health, better value. Dr. Robbin Dick is an industry thought leader who has devoted his career to making healthcare better. This patient-centered "playbook" provides healthcare leaders with proven strategies and practical process improvement tools for redesigning patient flow and capacity management in ways that can deliver a consistently exceptional patient care experience with greater efficiency and reliability."

Mark C. Clement,
President and CEO, TriHealth System

"The book provides a map for hospital leaders in navigating the challenge of reducing length of stay and increasing throughput. The approaches are practical and directed to increasing quality of care. The book belongs on the bookshelf of every hospital leader who is charged with capacity management."

Kevin Casey, MD
President Rochester General Hospital at Rochester Regional Health

"Hospital Capacity Management manages to take a highly complex topic and simplify it to tangible and executable recommendations. As hospital leaders we continually looking for better ways to use our resources in a cost effective and efficient manner. This book certainly provides the backbone to achieve these goals."

Michael Cetta, MD, FACEP, FACHE
Chief of Integrated Acute Care,
US Acute Care Solutions

Hospital Capacity Management

Hospital Capacity Management

Insights and Strategies

Robbin Dick, MD, FACP
Robert Agness

Routledge
Taylor & Francis Group
A PRODUCTIVITY PRESS BOOK

First Edition published 2021
by Routledge
600 Broken Sound Parkway #300, Boca Raton FL, 33487

and by Routledge
2 Park Square, Milton Park, Abingdon, Oxon, OX14 4RN

Routledge is an imprint of the Taylor & Francis Group, an informa business

Library of Congress Cataloging-in-Publication Data

ISBN: 978-0-367-70860-3 (hbk)
ISBN: 978-0-367-70858-0 (pbk)
ISBN: 978-1-003-14828-9 (ebk)

Typeset in Garamond
by SPi Global, India

Table of Contents

Letter from the Author

I felt it important to at least mention the fact that a worldwide pandemic is currently in place. Today is April 1, 2020. As of today, there are over 800,000 cases of this infection and over 40,000 deaths. This will increase significantly over the next few months to infect and kill millions. In the United States alone, there are over 180,000 infections and close to 4,000 deaths as of today. The hospitals in the country are reaching maximal capacity and will exceed maximal capacity shortly. There is nothing really good to report out as this is not the components of capacity management that our book is focused on. To give an example, the United States currently has about 150,000 ventilators for patients. The expected need is 600,000 to 700,000 ventilators. I can only hope at the time of this writing that it does not become reality.

Other issues with this disease process are those who get extremely ill. Approximately 15% of infected patients will require hospitalization and of those about 5% will require ICU level of care. There are nowhere near the level of ICU beds in the country to manage that kind of volume. In addition, patients who end up in the ICU have an average LOS of 15 days, where your typical ICU patient's LOS is 3 days. This consumes ICU bed capacity very quickly and relinquishes it very slowly.

Current mechanisms to deal with this disaster have been the conversion of non-healthcare areas such as convention centers to temporary hospitals. In NYC, they are converting the Javits Center into a hospital, tapping the National Strategic Reserves for Personal Protective Equipment and ventilators, sending the Medical Hospital Ships Hope and Comfort to the east and west cost to assist with their 1,000 beds each, and instituting shelter in place orders for citizens, closing restaurants, bars, theaters, schools, and all sporting events. Although these are all helpful components, they are the same management practices that hospitals institute when they develop overcapacity. This reactive management will assist but in no way resolve this problem.

This is not the first or will be the last of pandemics. I was in medical school when HIV was found. I was managing a large ED when SARS hit and H1N1 in 2009. These were all deadly and difficult to manage but not even close to the current virus. There needs to be both a global and national plan to manage and contain further infectious agents which can threaten the existence of humanity. This will require cooperation, not isolation; transparency, not lies and hidden agendas; and the coordination by a task force of experts to develop preparation for the next pandemic.

Robbin Dick, MD, FACP

About the Authors

Robbin Dick, MD, FACP

I started my career working in the Emergency Department in 1988 and trained in Internal Medicine. This role served me well in developing concepts and principles around efficiency and process improvement. Developing the first recognized observation unit in NY State to improve ED efficiency in 1996 was the start of investing many years of my career in observation medicine and hospital capacity management. In 2003, I joined the University of Rochester Emergency Department and implemented and managed a 36-bed observation unit. In 2009, I had the opportunity to focus on the use of Lean Six Sigma concepts in Hospital Capacity management. As Vice President of Clinical Efficiency, I had the opportunity to develop new models of care delivery and integration. I was Director of Observation Services managing the Observation Service line for Medical Emergency Professionals across the state of Maryland from 2012 to 2015.

In 2016, our company joined USACS and I served as Chief of Observation Services for our company until October of 2018, developing a National Observation Service Line. Development included well-defined protocols, a robust teaching module based off of MKSAP, testing guidelines, a peer review process, electronic iPad patient satisfaction program, and National Oversite of the Observation Programs operational development. USACS currently has over 15 observation units with over 70,000 encounters yearly and is the largest observation program in the United States. Currently, my focus is on consultative services in Observation Medicine & Hospital Capacity Management.

Robert Agness, B.A.

Robert is an experienced professional in operational management. He received Lean Six Sigma training under Shingo Ztisu trainers at Eastman Kodak's Lean Institute early in his career. His role at Kodak involved the application of Lean Six Sigma principles restructuring and redesigning internal processes and facilities. Robert spent his last years at Eastman Kodak implementing a lean factory as Operations Manager of its Digital Graphics manufacturing site.

Robert brought his expertise in Lean Six Sigma methodologies and implementation to Rochester General Health Systems in 2007. There he educated the leadership, developed a Lean Six Sigma Black Belt program equivalent, and facilitated the redesign of patient flow in the Emergency Department, Radiology, Peri-Op, and Inpatient Care Units. He also has designed and implemented the system's Central Bed Management Department, effecting greater efficiency across numerous departments. He managed patient flow and capacity management for two of the system's hospitals, totaling 600 beds.

Robert is currently semi-retired and works part-time as a consultant in Hospital Capacity Management providing recommendations and assistance utilizing Lean Six Sigma training.

Introduction

It is highly likely that each of us will experience a visit to the local hospital as a patient. This is rarely a joyous occasion (childbirth excluded) but a visit due to some injury or illness which we are anxious to have evaluated and treated, and for many of us, the experience can be extremely frustrating and confusing. Among the many reasons for this is the fact that most hospital systems have developed over years and years with little thought given to standards and process. The result is a system which works differently from one place to the next, often with wide variability in effectiveness and efficiency. For many years, individuals within the healthcare system simply did the best with what they had, as they reacted to new challenges and the ever-changing realities of healthcare. Today, patients often wonder why things are the way they are in hospitals. Why do I have to wait so long in the emergency department to be seen? Why is there such variability among providers? Why can't I get tests I want done in a timely and efficient manner? Why do I wait so long for a bed if I need to be in the hospital? Why does it take the doctor so long to get to me and why do my questions get different answers from different people?

This book is intended to uncover why some of these perplexing problems exist. It also presents and discusses potential solutions, and hopefully, this book will increase the knowledge base around how hospitals function so that they may eventually function much better than they currently do.

Some may find the tone of portions of the book rather cynical. If one examines the volume of patients that are injured yearly, many of whom die in the process of receiving the healthcare they are trying to acquire, it's no wonder that a cynical tone may emerge [28].

First and foremost, it is necessary to remember that the mission of our healthcare system is to take care of patients. This has been forgotten at times, causing many of the issues we will be looking at in this book. And that brings us to hospital capacity management. While it may sound less than fascinating, this facet of healthcare management is absolutely central to the success or failure of a hospital, both in terms of its delivery of care and its ability to survive as an institution. Poor hospital capacity management is a root cause of long wait times, overcrowding, higher error rates, poor communication, low satisfaction, and a host of other commonly experienced problems. It is important enough that when it is done well, it can completely transform an entire hospital system.

Hospital capacity management can be described as optimizing a hospital's bed availability to provide enough capacity for efficient, error-free patient evaluation and treatment to meet daily demand. A hospital that excels at capacity management is easy to spot: no lines of people waiting, no patients in hallways or sitting around in chairs. These hospitals do not divert incoming ambulances to other hospitals. They have excellent patient safety records and efficiently move patients through their organization. They exist, but are sadly in the minority of American hospitals. The vast majority instead are forced to constantly react to their own poor performance. Often this results in the building of bigger and bigger institutions, which, instead of managing capacity, simply create more space in which to mismanage it. These institutions are failing to resolve the true stumbling blocks to excellent patient care, many of which you may have experienced firsthand in your own visit to your hospital. It is our hope that this book will provide a better understanding of the healthcare delivery system.

Chapter 1

Hospital Priorities

Little has been written about hospital capacity management recently. But, as we shall see, capacity management depends on hospital priorities, a subject that fewer experts are willing to tackle, at least in public. As hospitals feel the impact of Value versus Volume, their administrations are scrambling to adapt to this new model. Central to their success will be the ability to improve hospital bed utilization while maintaining a high level of care. In fact, patient-centered care is another popular topic of discussion, as new healthcare laws penalize poor performance across a variety of quality metrics.

But the patient, in reality, is rarely the focus of administrative planning. Instead, physicians, nurses, residents, and even administrators are given priority. Yet, in order to succeed, healthcare must be about the patient. As we look at new ways to adapt our healthcare system, this must be remembered.

More patients enter the hospital through the Emergency Department (ED) than anywhere else. It is the front door to the hospital, a busy hive of activity where patients, family, friends, and providers interact in large numbers before being admitted, transferred, sent home, or held for observation. The ED is often a breeding ground for creative, patient-centered solutions to capacity-management and patient care challenges—Why?—because it has to be (2, 3, and 4). No one can predict how many patients will enter the ED on any given day, or what their needs will be. Therefore, the ED must be flexible, and it must be efficient (1). If it is not, costs can run sky-high, and patient care can suffer. The pain of a poorly performing ED is felt quickly and sharply by any hospital and has often been the cause of new processes and creative new thinking. In short, the ED is a natural incubator for effective new approaches to providing efficient, effective healthcare.

This is probably why the ED is also a hotbed of metric analysis. The ED is more scrutinized, across a wider variety of performance measures, than any other area of healthcare: Door-to-Doctor Time, Left-Without-Treatment (LWOT) Rate, Diversion Hours, Length-of-Stay, Test Utilization Rate, Door-to-EKG Time, Door-to-Cath Lab Time, Door-to-Antibiotic Delivery, Provider Relative Value Units (RVUs) Per Hour, Patient Satisfaction, and many more. These metrics tell us a great deal about what's working—and what's not—in the ED. They exist because hospitals must stay profitable in order to continue to provide services.

However, hospitals measure performance, any resulting initiative is likely to be subject to the hospital's real priorities. Sure, there are many dedicated providers and administrators whose focus is on patient-centered care—but the reality is that institutional priorities exist which have less to do with patient care than with continued profitability. This reality brings us to the central role that hospital priorities have played—and will play—in shaping the healthcare system.

Though many institutions would deny they have such priorities, they all do.

Here they are:

1. First priority is always high-margin surgical cases
2. Second are high-margin cardiac cases

3. Third are usually transfers and directs for a tertiary care facility
4. Lower margin surgical cases are given about the same priority as transfers and directs
5. The very last priority is the Emergency Department.

As a direct result of these priorities, ED beds are often filled with patients who do not belong in the ED. These can be patients who require surgery like appendicitis, patients awaiting high-margin services in other departments like a hip fracture or simply ED patients awaiting admittance to the hospital. This approach to capacity management, which is entirely motivated by a hospital's need to profit, reduces bed space available for incoming ED patients. Often during the highest volume period of the day, the ED has the fewest number of beds available. This results in long wait times and patients getting frustrated and leaving without being seen by a doctor. This is why many EDs get creative, placing patients in hallways, placing a provider in triage, and generally coping as well as they can while higher margin electively scheduled patients are given priority. Clearly, if any one area of the healthcare system understands the impact of misplaced priorities—and their effect on capacity management—it is the Emergency Department.

One result of this pecking order for hospital beds is that the ED experiences a repeating pattern of capacity management problems tied to the booking of Operating Rooms, cardiology, and the Cath lab. Long wait-times and crowding on Monday and Tuesday are common. This is a direct result of high scheduled volumes on those days for surgery and cardiology. Wednesday and Thursday are lighter as scheduled operations taper off. Friday, which almost always sees low volumes in surgery and cardiology, allows the ED to decompress a little. Wait times shorten and the crowds thin out. Then, with the weekend, provider staffing shrinks and the volume of discharges from the hospital is cut in half. Monday comes and the cycle repeats. This really is not capacity management at all, but it's common in most hospitals. True capacity management anticipates the needs of the organization and adjusts and coordinates variables within the control of the hospital in order to provide optimal bed use for all patients.

One such approach, which has gained a great deal of interest, is called Leveling. This is the practice of spreading Operating Room and Cath lab schedules throughout the week, rather than loading them up on Monday and Tuesday. In theory, this simple solution should greatly ease some of the capacity management problems of the hospital. A lot of studies have focused on this. However, in practice, leveling rarely works. This is because surgeons and cardiologists tend to schedule based on their own individual needs or preferences—and they are so high on the hospital's priority list that no one actually forces them to adhere to leveling rules. So, cardiothoracic surgeons have their own Operating Rooms. If they're running at only 50% occupancy, no one seems to mind. Other specialty units exist, too, often with criteria so rigid that many patients cannot use them. This reality will only change when hospitals determine that the most important thing in the organization is the patient, not the most profitable providers. So, when the Emergency Department has 25 patients waiting for a bed at 3 pm in the afternoon on Tuesday has anyone decided to close the Operating Rooms, the Cath labs, refuse directs or transfers? Not on your life. Priorities drive capacity management. This impact on the ED cascades into the hospital proper with multiple negative impacts (Figures 1.1 to 1.3).

The graphs clearly demonstrate the deleterious effects of patients spending extended stays in the Emergency Department awaiting a bed. Each of these parameters has a significant negative financial impact on the organization.

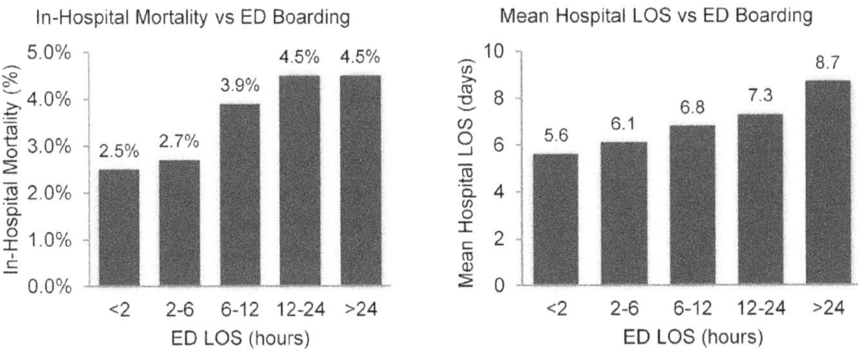

Figure 1.1 The impact increasing inpatient LOS in the ED can have on multiple variables. (Data drawn from a 187 bed Connecticut hospital and represent).

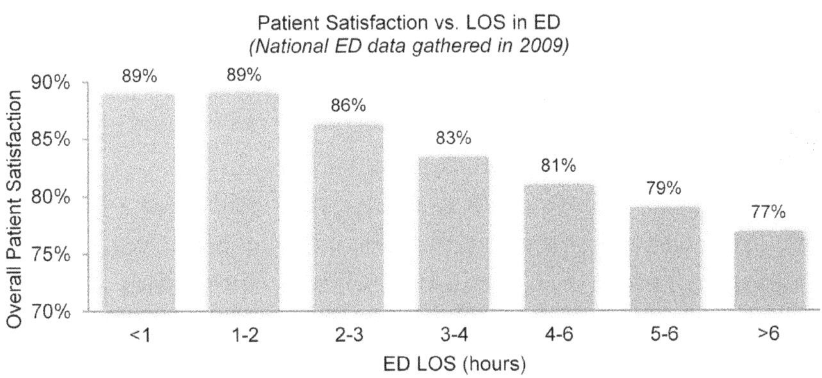

Figure 1.2 The impact increasing inpatient LOS in the ED can have on multiple variables. (Data drawn from a 187 bed Connecticut hospital and represent).

The longer patients stay in the ED awaiting a bed, the more significant these negative impacts become.

Understanding hospital priorities is therefore an essential first step, both for recognizing the problems hospitals face, and for developing workable solutions. Now it must also be understood that Hospitals did not design the current

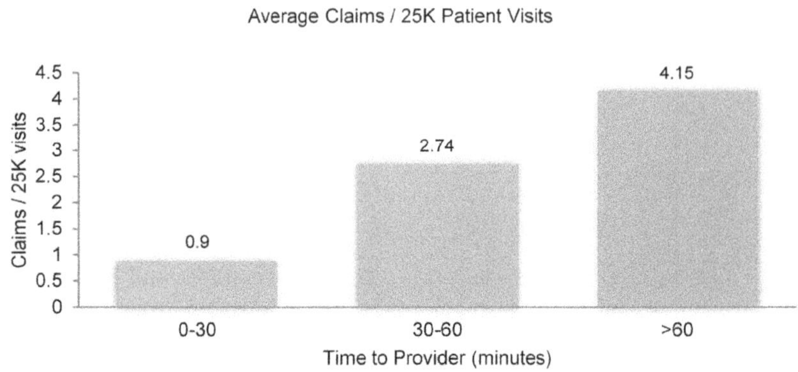

Figure 1.3 The impact increasing inpatient LOS in the ED can have on multiple variables. (Data drawn from a 187 bed Connecticut hospital and represent).

reimbursement system for healthcare that exists in the United States. This process of priorities is a consequence of adapting to that reimbursement system so the hospital can be financially viable. If the reimbursement system were changed, I suspect priorities would change as well.

The body of this book is comprised of real-world problems, and many proposed solutions, all of which were designed to better serve patients. So, without further ado, let's get started.

Chapter 2

Bed Assignment

This component of capacity management sets the pulse of the entire hospital, affecting every patient and every department from minute to minute, yet is often poorly managed. I have been amazed over the years at how many people desire the position of bed assigner. Nurses, Surgeons, Private Internists, Hospitalists, ED providers, and even Hospital Administrators at some point in time want to assign beds to patients. They often have no idea, however, how their decisions will affect ED wait times, Operating Room and Cath lab needs, and the flow of non-ED patients throughout the hospital, to name just a few factors that need to be considered. Yet bed assignment has far-reaching effects.

Many think that bed assignment is a simple task. In theory it should be. A bed is available, and the patient gets assigned. There are certain constraints—sex, semi-private versus private, isolation issues, acuity, telemetry, and specialty needs. All need to be taken into account to ensure that each patient goes to the right place and receives the proper care. But good capacity management demands that bed assignment be carefully considered and executed with fixed rules and guidelines:

Rule 1. Centralize bed assignment authority. All beds need to be assigned by a centralized authority—and no one else. Patients cannot be moved without a reason. Patients cannot be assigned by others. All discharges must quickly and accurately be handed over to environmental services for bed cleaning then immediately handed back to bed assignment. I can recall an analysis of environmental services staffing on the evening shift. Beds vacated by discharged patients at 5 pm were not being cleaned until 1 or 2 am. All the data said that there was sufficient staffing. Drilling down, we discovered that nursing staff had decided to transfer patients from one bed on their unit to another bed on the same unit, for multiple reasons, without contacting bed assignment. This was being done so frequently that it consumed 1/3 of the environmental staff that was allocated to clean beds for discharged patients. Thus, the need for rule 1 (Figure 2.1).

Rule 2. Use Non-clinical staff to do bed assignment. Set the rules and parameters on when and where patients can go and let them do their job. Nurses tend to look through clinical content to assign just the right bed. This wastes time and energy while producing no better results than non-clinical staff. The main reason clinical staff are involved at all is that there is an idea that bed assignment

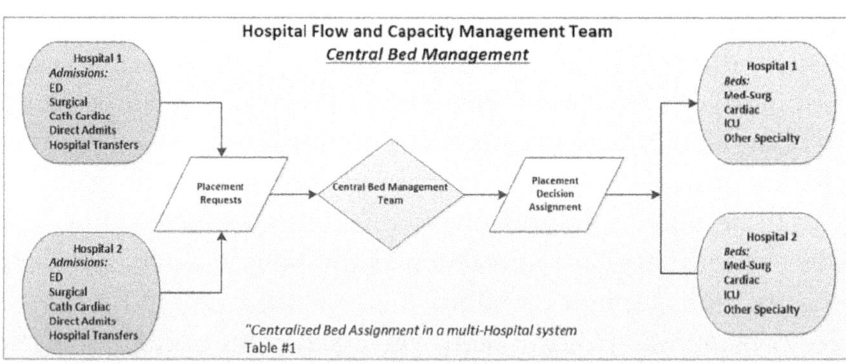

Figure 2.1 Flow chart diagramming Central Bed Group.

provides a clinical report on the patient to the accepting unit. This is not only inappropriate, but also dangerous since the true clinical status of a patient can rarely be gleaned from reviewing the chart, not to mention that care handoffs need to be done by the current care provider (where they are) and the receiving care provider. Bed assignment simply provides the proper location based on specific patient attributes like sex, isolation, telemetry, acuity, and specialty needs.

Rule 3. Provide a mechanism of escalation. When problems arise, the bed assignment staff needs help. Assistance with inadequate telemetry availability, limits on private room use, prevention of patient movement within the hospital, all can have a significant impact on bed assignment and timely patient placement.

Rule 4. Provide priorities and establish mechanisms to maintain them. Priorities for bed assignment need to be linked to the needs of the sickest patients in the organization, wherever they may be. Those patients requiring ICU level of care, whether in the ED, Post Anesthesia Care Unit (PACU), floor, or another facility needing to transfer the patient, would have the highest priority. It has been demonstrated that patients requiring this level of care have a lower mortality rate and suffer the fewest complications the quicker they are placed in the intensive care unit [5].

Bed Assignment Priorities

Priority 1: Sickest First-ICU. All hospitals should prioritize the sickest patients. Most of these cases enter the hospital through the ED and are often quickly transferred to a special intensive care unit. This transfer itself can be a failure point, as delays and miscommunication have been shown to raise mortality rates [29].

In general, hospitals should use a "bed ahead" policy, in which an ICU bed is always kept available. If a hospital fills all its ICU beds, the ICU needs to have already identified the next eligible patient for transfer out of the ICU. This will prioritize ICU patients for transfer, thus freeing up a bed.

A key aspect of ICU bed assignment is communication between the ICU and the bed assignment authority. A single point of contact, such as an assigned nurse who fields all transfer requests, can cut through delays and speed transfers in and out of the ICU. In many cases, a few moments can mean the difference between life and death—which is why these patients receive the highest priority. We'll discuss problems and process improvements around the ICU later on in this book.

Priority 2: Post-Surgical Patients. These patients are recovering from surgery and usually have specialty needs related to their procedures. Time spent in the PACU should be limited to avoid backing up an Operating Room. Operating costs for these rooms can exceed $1000 per h, making such a backup financially disastrous [6].

Numerous factors often contribute to poor performance here. In hospitals running extremely high occupancy, there is the tendency to back-fill every available bed with patients admitted through the Emergency Department. This results in specialty surgical beds filled with medical patients admitted through the ED when the hospital census is lower on the weekend, then on Monday require their movement off the surgical floor to an available medical floor when available. This approach wastes resources, time, and money. Better options include relocating nursing staff from the specialty areas to the ED to care for admitted patients, clustering admitted patients in a portion of the ED, and prioritizing these patients for disposition and discharge. Providers should focus their rounds, both in the ED and the hospital floor, on patients who might be discharged, freeing up beds and decompressing the hospital before noon, when the ED, PACU, and Cath lab fill up again. Placing specialty patients incorrectly is also a common problem. Specialty patients require specialty regions within the hospital proper. A medical unit is unlikely to have the specialty equipment to care for an orthopedic patient, for example. Unless placed correctly, specialty patients cause additional movements and wasted resources.

Poor surgical scheduling is also quite common, and can be extremely difficult to resolve, as we will discuss in more detail later on. Scheduling complex cases requiring an inpatient surgical bed early in the day places additional strain on a system with very high occupancy. I remember once suggesting to our surgeons that it would be better for bed utilization to perform complex surgical cases later in the day and elective outpatient cases earlier. This would result in more timely discharges and free up beds. The response I got was "I do my best work in the morning." I was unsure whether this meant that if I need surgery to make sure it was scheduled in the morning or that patients receiving later surgery were getting suboptimal surgical care. Needless to say, there was no enthusiasm to embrace this idea.

The good news is that there are quite a few steps hospitals can take to improve bed availability for PACU patients:

(a) Reserve beds for patients the night before surgery so there is immediate bed availability and a smooth transition from the PACU to the designated floor.
(b) Prepare a list of surgeries scheduled for the following week. Know exactly what to plan for and determine if bed needs will be met.
(c) Enact a leveling policy. As discussed above, most surgeries are elective and scheduled weeks ahead, presenting an opportunity to limit artificial variability of bed use [7]. This is a complex and difficult process to implement, however, and has met with much resistance due to its impact on provider lifestyles.

(d) Bring in OR cases the night before to prep for their case if beds are available. This is an excellent and customer friendly option.

(e) A 7-day weekly surgical scheduling policy would be of significant benefit but, as with leveling, will meet stiff resistance. I remember one time our team was doing a Capstone project with one of the Universities in town. The project was to determine the flow of patients through the organization and highlight when the hospital reached maximum capacity and would go on divert. The big day came, and we gathered in the auditorium to watch the computer demonstration that the students had worked on for months. The hospital was a 528-bed facility and the program had little figures moving continuously about the hospital. In the corner was a Bar that would move up and down to indicate hospital occupancy. When it reached maximum capacity, it would turn Red. We watched for quite a while and it never turned Red. I asked the students if they could remove beds from the program and run it again. They said yes and took 100 beds out, still no Red bar. Then another 100 and finally after removing 250 beds the Red bar showed up continuously. We asked a simply question of why this could be. Well, it seems when the students loaded all the data into the computer program and ran the program, they assumed the hospital functioned in the same manner 7 days a week. It was an excellent demonstration on the amount of excess capacity that exists in hospitals with their current Monday through Friday mindset.

(f) Schedule outpatient surgical cases early in the day and cases requiring an inpatient bed later in the day. This approach provides breathing room for the system to discharge patients and make beds available for the patients that need them.

Many of these approaches are discussed in more detail below. These cases will heavily impact hospital profitability and are therefore high on the priority list.

Priority 3: Post-Cath Patients. A majority of Cath procedures with interventions, Pacers, EP studies, and others are now considered outpatient only procedures and are expected to be discharged without utilization of an inpatient bed. However, patients who experience complications such as chest pain, bleeding, or an arrhythmia will require bed placement in an area with telemetry. Most of these cases could and should be leveled through proper scheduling. Otherwise, they will cause much movement and manipulation as beds are needed.

Most post-Cath procedure patients will need to be managed in an environment other than inpatient beds in the future. This will be driven by reimbursement, as insurers will want to avoid higher inpatient rates, as well as by ongoing improvements in interventional procedures and their safety. This patient population will likely be managed with Cath holding areas in the future.

Priority 4: Transfers and Directs. Many facilities provide services which are not available at outlying institutions. This is especially true of Trauma centers. Patients requiring specialty intervention often cannot be diverted elsewhere simply because there is nowhere else to send them—even if the receiving hospital is overcrowded and short on beds. In these situations, the patient gets the care needed regardless of the status of the receiving hospital. This is a good example of patient-centered care—but presents a real challenge to bed assignment (Figure 2.2).

When Emergency Departments are overwhelmed and a large volume of admissions are awaiting beds, hospitals begin to consider refusing non-emergent transfers from other facilities. In theory, these patients are already in hospital and require no special services, so a stressed hospital should

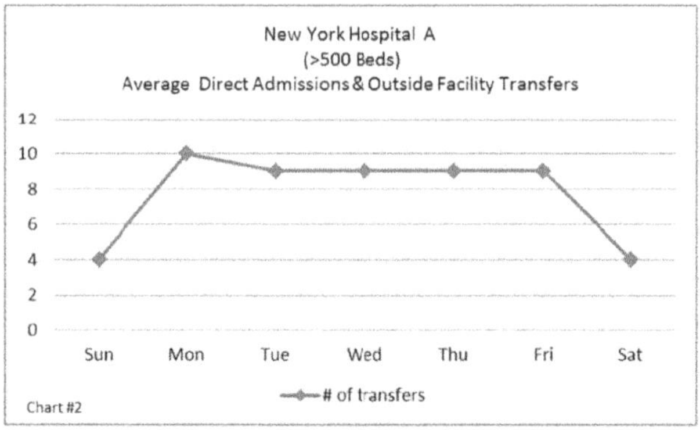

Figure 2.2 Anticipated daily new admissions from Primary Care Physicians, Surgeons, and Out of Network Facilities.

refuse the transfer in order to prevent problems with overcrowding. In practice, competition for patients from smaller outlying facilities drives administrations to find ways to take these patients anyway, even when the ED is stressed. This can cause the placement of more patients into an already overcrowded Emergency Department. Centralized bed assignment becomes crucial—and should have the benefit of clear direction from the administration and the administration must reach consensus on when to stop taking transfers.

Today, the majority of non-emergent transfers and directs occur on Monday through Friday, as seen in the graph above, a fact which indicates that administrations could also consider weekend transfers as a means to improve capacity management.

Priority 5: Emergency Department Admissions. It is an unfortunate fact that the ED has the lowest priority for admitted patient bed assignment in every organization I have ever seen. There are multiple reasons for this:

(1) Closure of the Operating Room or the Cath lab to free up beds is financially devastating
(2) Leaving patients in either the PACU or Cath lab will result in excessive cost in each area

(3) The Emergency Department already has the skill sets to care for admitted patients so there really is no rush.
(4) There are always doctors in the Emergency Department to handle a patient problem
(5) An overwhelmed ED is perceived to be less costly than an overwhelmed Operating Room or Cath lab, despite having some significant costs of its own.

In fact, patients who leave without receiving treatment (LWOTs) cost around $400 in lost revenue each, diversions (sending patients elsewhere) result in over $2,000 an hour of lost hospital revenue and low patient satisfaction results in lost revenue as patients take their hip, knee and other elective procedures elsewhere and encourage family and friends to do the same. Also, CMS now penalizes hospitals with poor patient satisfaction scores and rewards those who score well, providing additional financial pressure to improve in this area [8, 9].

Even before we delve further into the realities of capacity management, it is easy to understand how the many pressures and challenges faced by Emergency Departments has forced them to get creative and find ways to cope with often difficult conditions. This creativity is at the root of many of the proposed solutions we offer in this book, many of which are proven to be effective in real hospitals operating today.

While our approach to bed assignment does not attempt to shift hospital priorities, it will help relieve pressure on the ED, and can be implemented alongside all of the other programs we suggest later on, which, in turn, should help reduce the pressure on this highly sensitive area of our healthcare system even further. The result, in the end, will be better service and care for all patients, regardless of where they stack up in a hospital's list of priorities.

Chapter 3

Inpatient and Outpatient

The complexity of hospital capacity management does not end with bed assignment. Another factor to consider when admitting patients is that they must be categorized as either an inpatient or outpatient. Categorizations vary with insurance policies, Medicare rules, changing medical needs, and various other factors. And for both the patient and the medical facility, mistakes can be costly, causing higher out-of-pocket expenses, potentially for both the patient and the hospital. To understand how the classification and admission process actually works—and where it sometimes breaks down—it is necessary to look more closely at how Surgery, Cardiology and the Emergency Department each classify and handle admissions, as each area handles its patients in different ways.

Surgery

Surgical patients come from the ED, the floor, Transfers from another facility or have been scheduled for an elective procedure. A list of scheduled electives is generally available a week or more in advance (Figure 3.1).

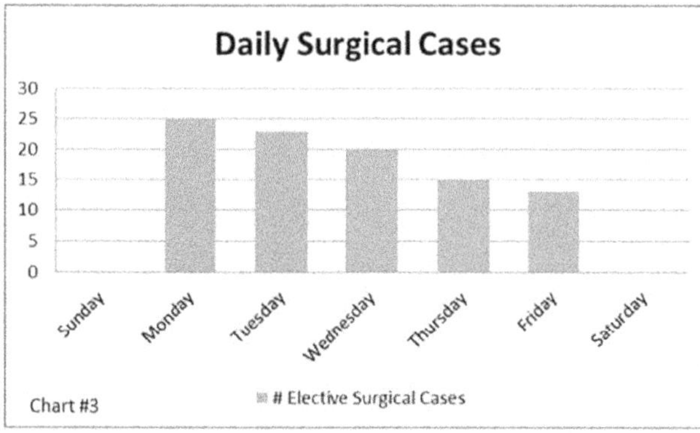

Figure 3.1 Reference from a Western New York 500-bed hospital.

Commercial insurers often determine whether an elective procedure is categorized as in-patient or outpatient through their approval process. Medicare also influences whether a procedure is considered inpatient or outpatient. Medicare publishes a yearly updated list on the CMS.gov website of which surgical procedures are deemed outpatient only.

But what is the definition of inpatient versus outpatient Surgical procedures? In practice, it varies from one insurer to the next. The most used definition is that: "...if a procedure is done without complications and the patient is expected to be discharged after their recovery period then they are considered an outpatient." The sticky part here is "without complications." What if the patient has refractory vomiting, hypoxia, hypotension, or any other issues? A surgeon is likely to make a clinical decision to keep that patient in the hospital. This type of unanticipated short-term hospital stay is what many facilities refer to as "extended recovery." It is still categorized as an outpatient stay. The hospital now needs additional beds to manage the short stays of this unanticipated group of outpatients. Although the number of these patients can vary, some extended recovery cases are actually scheduled, as surgeons sometimes know full well that the patient is not going home after the procedure and will need an inpatient bed and the hospital will be denied inpatient reimbursement.

The reason for this is the difficulty in obtaining prior authorization by a commercial insurer for an inpatient surgical procedure. There are significant hurdles to overcome, often involving time on the phone and filling out paperwork, and there is seldom time to build a case and win authorization for the inpatient stay. Subsequently, patients are placed in elective outpatient status on the Operating Room schedule. This impacts overall bed management for the organization when an unanticipated number of patients thought to be going home now need a bed.

Managing the Operating Room population starts with these elective procedures but gets more complex when the ED surgical cases like appendicitis or cholecystitis are taken into account. Both, if done laparoscopically without complications, are considered outpatient procedures, but if done by open incision are classified as inpatient. This has serious future repercussions with the utilization of robotic surgery and the significant increase in laparoscopic procedures. There has been a profound increase in surgical cases being done as an outpatient. I recently read of cardiothoracic bypass surgery being done laparoscopically. In the future, these cases may transition to ambulatory outpatient surgical suites with significant financial consequences to hospitals margins.

Then there are surgical specialties. The hospital clusters groups of similar-type patients in specialized areas for a lot of very good reasons. They all require the same specialty skills, specialty equipment, and specialty services like physical therapy for the orthopedic floor. Keeping these patient types together aids in their efficient movement through the system and ensures they all access the services they need.

The units themselves are a challenge for bed assignment. Procedures which send patients to any given specialty unit are not leveled during the week, so beds are occupied in waves. A high volume of Orthopedic cases on Monday and Tuesday then reduced caseload Wednesday through Friday with virtually zero cases scheduled Saturday and Sunday. Then a full unit on Wednesday but deficient volume for the unit on Thursday or Friday. This creates significant bed utilization problems for bed assignment. Most places prefer to send only orthopedic cases to the orthopedic floor, but if additional beds on the orthopedic unit are available, they are assigned to "stable medical patients." This results in varying numbers of orthopedic patients occupying the unit, which is backfilled with a mix of medical cases. On the weekend, when a significant number of orthopedic cases have left, ED medical admissions are placed in the unit's available beds. Then on Monday morning, we have an orthopedic unit functioning as a medical unit (Figure 3.2).

Suddenly, the operating room, which is now very busy, is desperate to move all the medical patients off their specialty unit because it's orthopedic Monday.

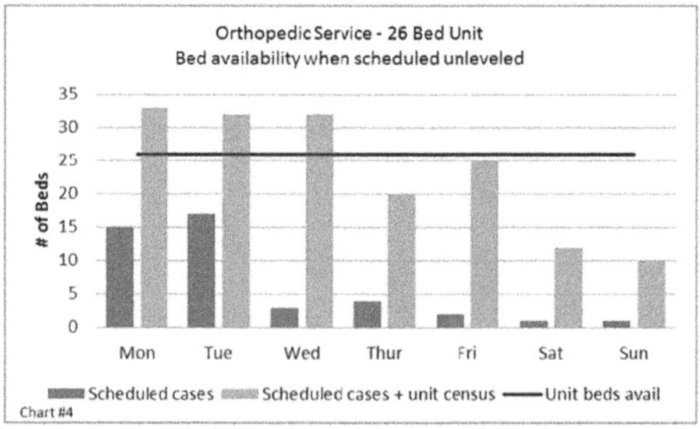

Figure 3.2 Bed shortage of an Orthopedic unit when the number of beds and Length of Stay (LOS) of Ortho cases are not used to implement a leveled surgical schedule. Shows impact on patients/unit of an unconstrained Surgical Schedule.

Cardiology

This area functions much like the surgical arena. Portals of entry again are the ED, Transfers, floor patients, and direct elective admissions. Some facilities do not offer full cardiac services such as catheterizations and EP studies. Those that do usually want the patients in a specific area for the same reasons surgical specialty units were created. Cardiology has come a long way from the 10-day LOS for acute Myocardial Infarction which was common 30 years ago. Today, it is common for a patient undergoing a significant interventional procedure to stay less than 48 h. Elective procedures that require intervention are considered now to be outpatient procedures similar to the extended recovery cases that surgery manages. Here again, we find the use of inpatient beds for patients considered to be in the outpatient world. Complications such as chest pain, arrhythmias, or bleeding can clearly move a patient into an inpatient status, but this is a minority of these patients.

The same issues described for surgery happen with cardiac catheterizations. Since elective scheduled procedures are the lion's share of cardiac procedures done, there is again a Monday through Friday scheduling issue—Heavy Monday and Tuesday and light Thursday and Friday. This non-leveled schedule results in the cardiac specialty floor again being utilized by ED medical admissions on the weekend and screams from the unit to "move these medical patients" come Cath-lab Monday (Figure 3.3).

Cardiology is unique in the management of potential cardiac patients because they have two types of outpatients to manage. The elective outpatient procedural patients and the "observation" patients. Observation is a status created by CMS to manage patients who don't have an immediately identified acute medical problem but whose presentation may evolve into one. There are a number of cardiac-type cases that fall

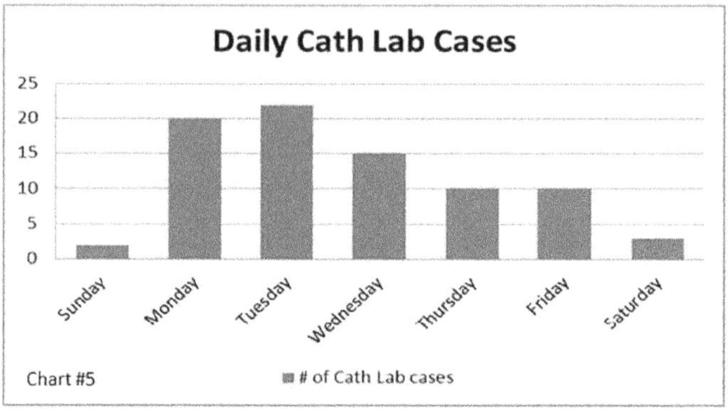

Figure 3.3 Unconstrained Cath Schedule leads to front loading of cases Monday through Wednesday, resulting in "non-cardiac" occupancy of the Cardiac floor Thursday through Sunday.

into this category including but not limited to chest pain, syncope, congestive heart failure and arrhythmias.

So how is the observation status identified and why is it important to bed assignment? Here again is a patient whose services are paid for on an outpatient reimbursement structure even though the patient may well be in an inpatient bed. The majority of these "observation" admissions come from the ED. One would think that this would be of benefit in optimizing the use of the cardiac specialty unit and maintaining its occupancy but remember the primary priority patient for the unit is the post cardiac procedure patient—not the ED admission. Many of these observation cardiac patients are simply scattered to the winds in most hospitals resulting in significant loss of efficiency and increases in LOS. We'll take a closer look at "observation" patients and their care in a later section.

Chapter 4

Emergency Department

The Emergency Department (ED) is an area of high natural variability. There is no predicting how busy a particular day or night may be. However, volume per hour curves exist which can help the ED know when to expect an increase. It is usual to be relatively slow between 7 am and 11 am, then a bit of an increase until 1 pm, then becoming very high volume consistently until about 12 mid-night or 1 am, and then rapidly ratcheting down to minimal levels until the am and the cycle repeats (Figure 4.1).

This cycle is fairly common 7 days a week, 365 days a year with some minor exceptions. This is important because it presents an opportunity. The period of lower volume presents a chance to decompress the ED before the next rush of incoming patients. This should be the time to clear the ED of any and all admissions who are still occupying its beds. But on many days, there's a problem. While the ED has spent Sunday, for example, admitting patients at a normal pace, on Monday morning, they have no beds to send them to. These patients, often called boarders, become admissions with no assigned inpatient bed occupying space in the ED. This occurs often when the higher priority Operating Room and

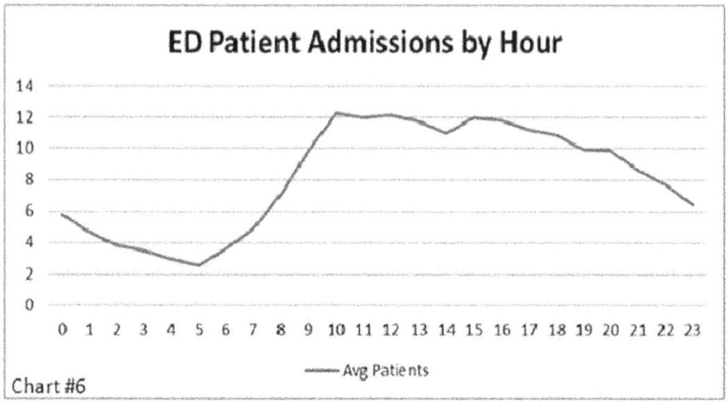

Figure 4.1 Average hourly admissions of a Western New York hospital with visits greater than 100k.

Cath lab, along with Directs and Transfers, take available inpatient beds, leaving ED admits in the ED. Obviously this scenario occurs predominantly in those institutions which have high bed occupancy utilization but even in lower occupancy models the process can be almost identical.

The ED is a complex admission environment admitting virtually all patient types:

(1) Acute Medical Inpatients
(2) Acute Surgical Inpatients
(3) Extended Recovery Surgical Patients (Outpatients)
(4) Urgent or Emergent Cath Lab Patients
(5) Medical Observation Patients

Of these five "admission" types, only two are considered to be pure inpatients. The determination of "Inpatient," "Outpatient," or "Observation" status varies by payer and patient type. Commercial insurance, Medicaid, and Medicare all vary. Medical patients are routinely given observation status, while elective surgical and Cath patients rarely meet the designation of observation but rather fall into the extended recovery arena.

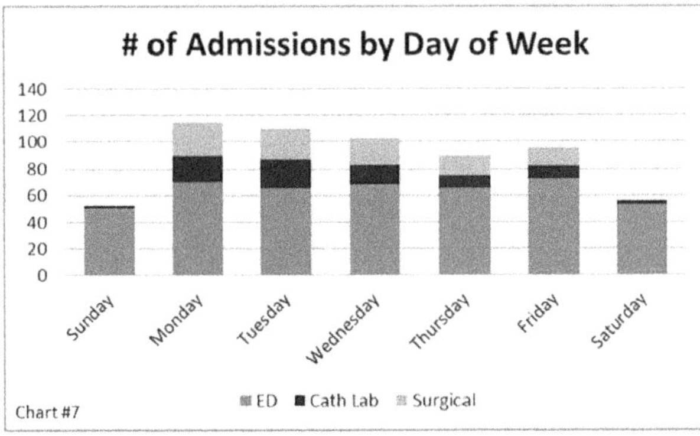

Figure 4.2 Total admissions for all demand streams by day of week for a Western New York hospital.

This can make assignment and location of ED admissions extremely difficult if the primary desire is to optimize bed capacity and resources. The reason for this is the variability of acuity of patient types and the impact these patient types can have on associated staffing ratios. Placing outpatients in inpatient beds wherever they are available will impact the overall volume of patients cared for by both nursing and provider staff (Figure 4.2).

Complex acute medical and surgical cases require smaller ratios for nursing, with the classic example being ICU in which patient to nurse ratios rarely exceed 2:1. With ratios like that, it only takes a few poorly placed patients to create a significant staffing problem.

Observation Care

The status of observation first occurred back in the 1980's when it was recognized that a subset of patients didn't neatly fit into the new Diagnosis-Related Group (DRG) reimbursement program. Then, in 2001, Medicare changed the way observation status was defined and paid for. At first, due to some abuse of the system which resulted in excessive billing,

Medicare completely removed the status. This abuse was predominantly hospitals billing for observation services for any patient in the hospital not classified as an inpatient. This included post-operative outpatient surgical cases, outpatient procedural cases, etc. This elimination of Observation status did not last that long because hospitals then started to bill any short-term medical patient as inpatients causing additional issues for Medicare. Then, it resumed observation, but with tight limitations, only allowing patients with chest pain, asthma, or CHF.

In 2003, Medicare again allowed all medical patients to be eligible for observation services, but this time with certain caveats:

(1) Patients placed into Observation from the ED had to be a level 4 or 5 acuity (patients that require hospitalization from the ED are given an acuity rating between 1 and 5 which identifies the severity of the patient condition and the intensity of services the patient needs).
(2) Observation patients required separate documentation for HPI, PMH, SH, FH, and meet requirements for a specific number of organ systems reviewed (ten) and physical exam findings (eight) documented.
(3) Different billing codes were developed for the professional fee component related to observation and the facility fee became a blended rate between the ED and the hospital facility fee. In hospitals, there are both professional fees and facility fees. I was seeing a patient who went on a lengthy rant about all the different bills he kept getting. The patient had previously been hospitalized as an observation patient and was getting separate bills for everything done. A facility bill for the hospital, a professional bill from the ED Doctor, a facility bill for an x-ray and an EKG, a professional bill for reading the x-ray and EKG and on and on.

It is understandable why patients have such a fit over the way healthcare is billed and paid for in the United States.

(4) Documentation had to be provided on an ongoing basis to identify why the patient continued to be placed in Observation status.
(5) Patients would be billed according to Medicare Part-B, outpatient regulations.
(6) Observation should be considered for patients whose disposition decision would be made in less than 24 h and not to exceed 48 h in duration—in October of 2014 a more recent implementation of this has become what is now known as the "2-mid-night rule "by Medicare [10].
(7) Patients deemed ineligible for Observation are patients where an elective procedure was ordered for convenience of the patient, patients receiving elective blood transfusions and patients who required a "social" admission.

Most hospitals have dealt with this concept of observation in what can best be described as a scatter-bed approach. Observation patients are often placed into any available inpatient bed that is currently empty, taking into account attributes such as sex, isolation needs, and telemetry. This seat-of-the-pants approach has a number of consequences both positive and negative.

From a hospital's perspective, the obvious positives of a typical "scatter bed" approach to assigning observation patients are that it costs nothing to set up and requires no change to staffing models. In these hospitals, Observation patients are generally viewed no differently than inpatients.

But the negatives are significant. First, there is almost always an increased Length of Stay (LOS) with scatter-bed observation. Then, because inpatients generate more revenue than observation patients, these hospitals lose revenue by decreasing inpatient bed availability. Also, they learn that they do need to adopt more expensive staffing ratios to handle the new mix of patients. There are also costs associated with the new outpatient reimbursement model of observation. In January of 2016, Medicare developed a new outpatient code C-APC 8011. This Comprehensive Ambulatory Classification code is now a bundled reimbursement for Medicare Fee for service patients. So regardless what tests, labs, etc., are done and how long the patient remains in the hospital, Medicare pays a flat bundled rate to the hospital of approximately $2400.00. This now behooves hospitals to do less in a quicker time frame to avoid taking a financial loss on these patient types. The one positive benefit is that Medicare Beneficiaries have a fairly good idea of their co-pay for an observation stay.

One of the keys to capacity management is to cluster patients similar in type. Placing them in one area with established protocols, skilled staff, and identified metrics can have a significant impact on LOS, quality of care and, not surprisingly, patient satisfaction [36]. This approach is used in cardiology, OB/GYN, Pediatrics, Cardio-thoracic surgery, Orthopedics, and other specialties. Taking a large group of medical outpatients (Observation) and placing them in a defined area and providing them with a standard process can have a significant impact on capacity and bed management. It has other major benefits as well, which we'll look at later, the "scatter bed" placement of observation patients rarely has a net positive effect for the patients or for the hospital. We will take a more detailed look at this problem—and some real-world solutions, later on.

Determining Patients Level of Care

Hospitals are often penalized financially for incorrectly determining a patient's level of care. This level of care is basically a determination of whether the patient is in inpatient or outpatient status. The hospitals level of care determinations can be reviewed for mistakes. Many reviewers exist, such as the Recovery Audit Committee (RAC) and the Medicaid Audit Committee (MAC), and they can levy huge fines—and do so—if they determine that mistakes were made. Other reviewers such as the QIO (Quality Improvement Organization), review hospital cases for accuracy in level of care determination. Though the QIO's are designed for educational purposes, they do have the ability to refer hospitals for more stringent reviews with RAC auditors if the hospital has ongoing problems with medical necessity accuracy (Figure 4.3).

There are three primary portals of entry which require the presence of a reviewer to determine the patient's medical necessity and the type of location within the hospital where the patient would be best served: the Emergency Department, the Operating Room or PACU and the Cardiac Cath lab. In most institutions, this person is a care or case manager. Usually a registered Nurse with prior clinical experience and an ability to review documented data and use clinical decision making to cross reference with some type of guideline such as InterQual or Millimans [12, 13] (Figure 4.4).

Utilization of reviewers in the three portals of entry can vary. The majority of patients coming out of the Operating

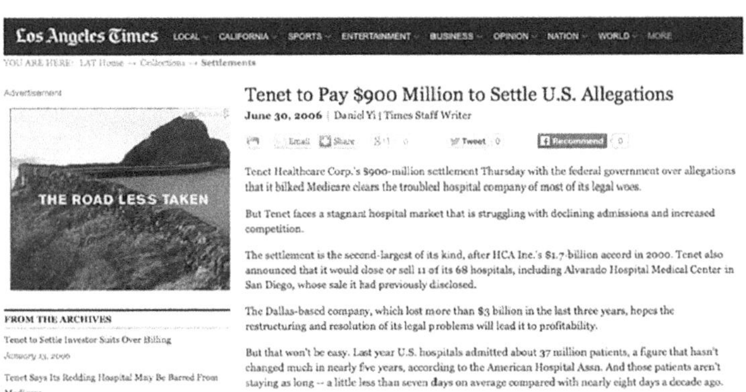

Los Angeles Times LOCAL CALIFORNIA SPORTS ENTERTAINMENT BUSINESS OPINION NATION WORLD MORE

YOU ARE HERE: LAT Home → Collections → Settlements

Advertisement

THE ROAD LESS TAKEN

Tenet to Pay $900 Million to Settle U.S. Allegations

June 30, 2006 | Daniel Yi | Times Staff Writer

Email Share Tweet 0 Recommend 0

Tenet Healthcare Corp.'s $900-million settlement Thursday with the federal government over allegations that it bilked Medicare clears the troubled hospital company of most of its legal woes.

But Tenet faces a stagnant hospital market that is struggling with declining admissions and increased competition.

The settlement is the second-largest of its kind, after HCA Inc.'s $1.7-billion accord in 2000. Tenet also announced that it would close or sell 11 of its 68 hospitals, including Alvarado Hospital Medical Center in San Diego, whose sale it had previously disclosed.

The Dallas-based company, which lost more than $3 billion in the last three years, hopes the restructuring and resolution of its legal problems will lead it to profitability.

But that won't be easy. Last year U.S. hospitals admitted about 37 million patients, a figure that hasn't changed much in nearly five years, according to the American Hospital Assn. And those patients aren't staying as long -- a little less than seven days on average compared with nearly eight days a decade ago.

FROM THE ARCHIVES

Tenet to Settle Investor Suits Over Billing

Tenet Says Its Redding Hospital May Be Barred From Medicare

Figure 4.3 Example where health care organizations are penalized.

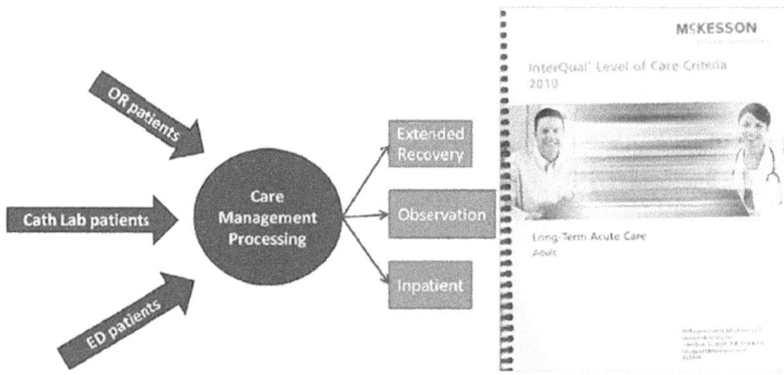

Figure 4.4 Care Management role in determining patient level of care.

Room and the Cath lab have had a predetermined status. The case manager's job here is to determine if that status has changed due to some complication or unexpected symptomatology associated with the procedure. The patients coming from these two portals are predominantly entering the hospital Monday through Friday as surgery and cardiac procedures are seldom scheduled on weekends and off-hours. Rare indeed is the institution that has moved to performing these procedures 7 days a week, 365 days a year.

Emergency Department Admissions

The Emergency Department is quite a different story. Here the complexities of review are much more important in acquiring the most correct level of care possible and getting the patient to the right location. The cost of not performing this process correctly can be significant in the form of lost revenue, fines or penalties, and a serious impact on the capacity management of the institution.

Patients whose criteria clearly fulfill the need for an acute inpatient admission are relatively straightforward. An example is the patient with a myocardial infarction, or a stroke documented on a CT scan or exam. Low-level patients are also relatively easy to determine. These cases, such as non-hypoxic asthma or chest pain with no acute concerns, meet none of the criteria for acute admission. But the gray area between these two groups includes many patients requiring more extensive review.

Of the patients who come into the ED and are then hospitalized, only about 20% have obvious diagnoses. Approximately 30% of ED Hospitalizations become observation patients. Many of these cases have symptoms which might be related to a serious condition but are not immediately life-threatening. Often a diagnosis is unclear. This is the classic chest pain patient in which the patient had symptoms but no indication of an acute problem such as a myocardial infarction, pulmonary embolus, pneumothorax, or aortic dissection. These patients often have an unremarkable initial work-up and no acute disorder, so they are placed somewhere in the hospital to undergo further diagnostic testing. For a suspected cardiac patient, this might require serial cardiac enzyme studies, putting the patient on telemetry, serial EKG's, and potentially provocative testing, all of which will take some time in the hospital.

These cases may require face-to-face interaction between the case manager and the ED provider in order to assess the most correct level of care. This becomes all important over the course of the next 24–36 h when patients not deemed eligible for acute inpatient status have to be reviewed on a daily basis to determine if that eligibility has now changed and the patient status upgraded to acute inpatient level of care (Figure 4.5).

This may also require contact with a commercial insurer for approval of an upgrade to inpatient level of care. The more robust the initial evaluation and determination is, the fewer re-reviews (rework) have to be done the next day and significant costs are saved as well as patients being placed in the proper location with their specific needs met.

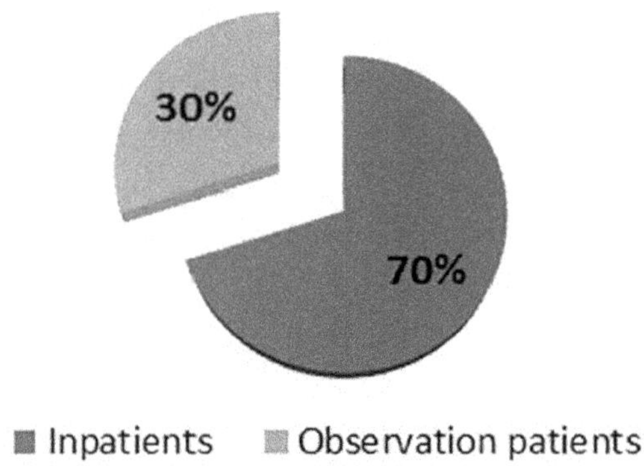

Figure 4.5 Average split between Inpatients and Observation Patients hospitalized from ED.

Other patients who have undergone treatment for known conditions, such as asthma, for example, may require additional ongoing treatment before they are stable enough to be discharged. These cases are also placed into observation status and must be assigned a bed in the hospital. The remaining 70% of Hospitalizations that come through the Emergency Department, are assessed as "acute inpatient" or "outpatient" cases for a variety of reasons. Patients requiring hospitalization through the ED are often in the early stages of a disease. Predicting where these patients are in the disease process, and therefore whether and when they may get sicker, is very difficult. A classic example is pneumonia or pyelonephritis. In their early stages, these diseases are notoriously difficult to predict. It is almost impossible to determine if the patient is likely to get sicker quicker. This can make an accurate assessment of "acute inpatient" or "outpatient" very difficult.

Hospitalizations through the ED usually come in waves, presenting a different type of challenge when assessing them. These hospitalizations come in boluses for several reasons, such as when an ED shift changes, causing providers to make a definitive decision of admit, discharge, or transfer. Lack of a decision results in signing the patient out to the oncoming provider and is something most ED providers try to avoid. In EDs that utilize demand level staffing, (having enough provider staff to manage high volume periods), high patient volumes can result in multiple providers making admission determinations in a short period of time. These waves of admissions can overwhelm a system's bed assigner, as well as any care managers assigned to determine levels of care in real-time.

It should not be assumed that an ED doctor is overly concerned about the correct determination of an "ED admission or Hospitalization." The decision the ED provider makes is whether or not the patient requires hospitalization. This is strictly about the care of the patient and does not enter into the realm of insurance categorization. Whether the patient has a serious illness, potentially serious illness or is simply an unsafe discharge, will drive the decision for hospitalization. Getting a busy doctor to participate in a level of care determination can be difficult because it can shift his or her focus from patient care and can be time-consuming. This presents a further challenge to accurate, timely, level-of-care determinations.

Some changes in status do occur. Observation patients may end up being upgraded to acute inpatients, usually due to the patient's condition worsening. This typically involves contacting commercial insurers to obtain an authorization or agreement that the patient's condition now warrants inpatient level of care. The patient is often completely unaware of this upgrade, though it can have a number of consequences related to payment responsibilities or eligibility for alternate care resources when the patient is discharged from the acute care facility.

If a Medicare patient was designated as an acute inpatient upon hospitalization, but a review determines that the patient should really be an observation patient, a compliance process, termed "code 44" is initiated. A series of tasks must be completed during the patient's hospitalization. The initial physician must document why the change occurred, a second provider must agree with the change in writing, the patient must be informed, both verbally and in writing, and a new order for the change of level of care must be written [11].

Finally, the many ED metrics in use can have an important role in timely decision making. Many ED providers have incentives based on performance metrics such as Door to Doc times, Door to Bedtimes, ED treat and release times, and ED admission LOS. The following figures demonstrate some of these metrics in graphical detail (Figures 4.6–4.8).

The importance of determining the appropriate level of care for patients has changed the way hospitals operate. They are penalized, unless they get it right from the moment a patient is admitted or hospitalized. Once admitted, frequent re-evaluations are made to determine if a change is required. These efforts are now central to hospital admitting policies and procedures. Since the ED generates the vast majority of non-predetermined cases, it has (or should) become the focus of efforts to improve performance in this area. One might think that any easy way around all this medical necessity

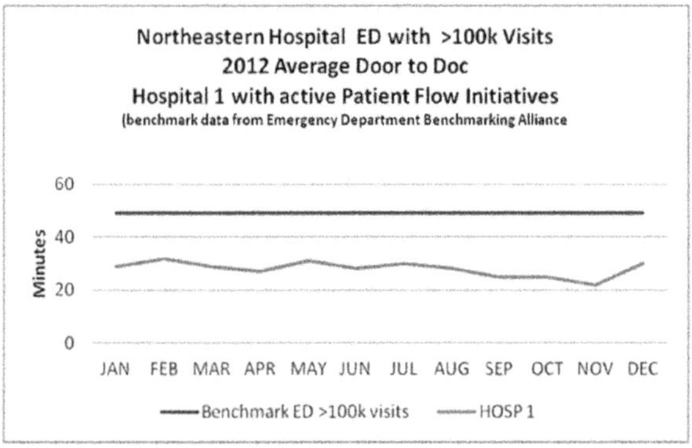

Figure 4.6 Improvements seen in large volume EDs when Patient Flow initiatives are implemented.

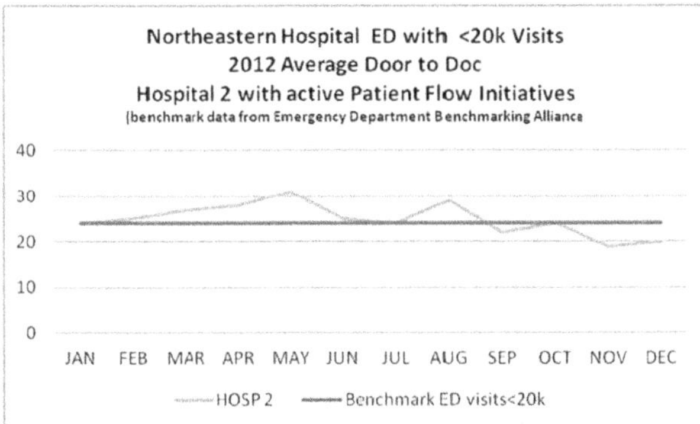

Figure 4.7 Improvements seen in smaller volume EDs when Patient Flow initiatives are implemented.

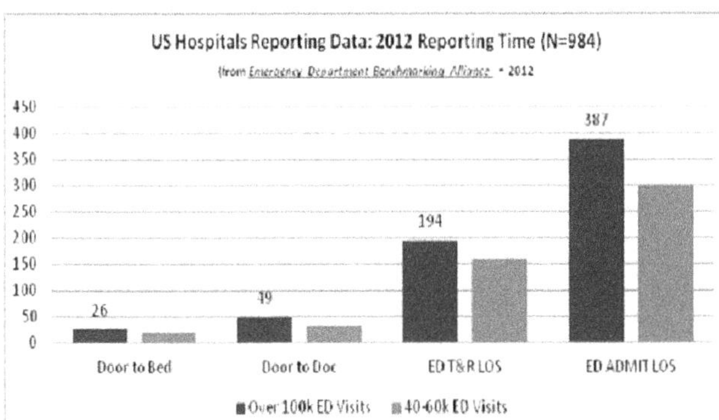

Figure 4.8 US Hospital average times for ED Patient Throughputs.

determination and level of care, is simply to make all the patients requiring hospitalization from the ED be initially placed in Observation status. Then if the patient gets sicker, the hospital can change the status to inpatient level of care. This type of decision making has consequences. The first is the impact of all hospitalized patients being placed in Observation status. This results in artificially reducing the LOS of Inpatients. This is important because Inpatient LOS is a contributor to the calculation of Case Mix Index (CMI). This index is utilized to determine payment by Medicare to the hospital and small fluctuations in this index can have serious financial repercussions. Artificially reducing LOS for the Medicare Inpatient population can reduce the hospitals CMI. The second issue is the additional resources necessary to review all hospitalizations for level of care changes if all patients are placed in Observation status initially instead of only the 30% of hospitalizations from the ED that would normally be reviewed. Once a level of care is determined, bed assignment must take place, but as we have already noted, this process has its challenges too.

Chapter 5

Types of Hospital Beds

Hospitals are constructed to suit the needs of their communities and to meet demand for services. Competition, population growth, economic conditions, and many other realities are considered carefully and then, as these factors change over time, the hospital must adapt to corresponding changes in demand. Not surprisingly, hospital capabilities vary widely. A hospital may or may not offer specialty procedures, complex care, trauma care, academic programs, and many other services. Every hospital's physical space is a reflection of the services it provides, its priorities, and its continual adaptation to shifting needs and demands. The hospital's beds, which both define and limit patient populations, can be of several types, and can, play a major role in how well a hospital meets the needs of its community and its own need to be financially healthy.

In terms of capacity management, a hospital's size and its number of beds is extremely important. It can have too many beds, costing money and impacting efficiency. It has been known for hospitals to mothball beds that see little use. Too few and it may fail to meet patient needs, while facing heavy construction costs as it expands to meet demand. Finding the sweet spot of optimal utilization and efficiency is a major challenge. Beyond how many beds are needed, every hospital must consider what types of beds to offer, how to arrange them, how to move patients from one to another, and many other details, all of which has an impact on its success and on patient experiences upon entering the hospital. To understand these factors, and how they affect hospital performance, it is necessary to take a closer look at the beds themselves and how they fit into a hospital's service model. This particular issue became front and center during the Covid-19 pandemic in 2020. Hospital beds were reallocated almost daily to try and keep up with ICU bed demand.

ICU Intensive Care Beds

This bed is designed to cater to the sickest and most complex of hospital patients. The beds will normally have all the required high-level equipment to support ventilators, arterial lines, oxygen, suction, dialysis, and telemetry needs. These beds are almost always private, and their staffing usually has a 2:1 patient to nurse ratio. Intensive care beds are deployed in a variety of ways by different hospitals. Some hospitals have multiple specialty ICUs, isolating areas such as Surgical, Medical, Cardiothoracic, and Vascular. Each of these might have its own dedicated staff while managing only a select type of patient. Rarely do multiple ICU types cross-utilize beds or staff. This makes them highly inefficient for overall bed utilization. These units often compound their inefficiency with uneven elective procedure scheduling, which can further lower bed occupancy while raising the costs of staffing.

Hospitals also vary when it comes to determining who requires ICU level of care. Most organizations have specific criteria that require placement in an ICU bed. Examples are acute ventilator patients, arterial lines, femoral lines, certain IV drugs, such as vasopressors, or certain anti-arrhythmic agents. Although this list seems reasonable, there are many times strict adherence to these regulations places patients in the ICU who do not really need to be there. A patient, for example, may be getting IV Cardizem for atrial fibrillation rate control. This patient may be perfectly stable and could be managed in an alternative telemetry environment, but hospital regulation requires placement in the ICU because of the Cardizem. Hospitals therefore vary on their ICU placement criteria.

Many hospitals devote 20% of their bed space to the ICU. Some make ICU beds as high as 40% of their total bed availability [14]. A significant factor in determining this is the length of stay of patients in the ICU setting, because the longer the LOS, the more beds will be required. Frequent rounding, aggressive therapy, defined weaning protocols, and linkage to palliative care are necessities which have a significant impact on length of stay and proper unit sizing.

ICU beds are crucial to capacity management. Because priority is always given to the sickest patients, an ICU bed must always be available for the next patient requiring this level of care. Therefore, bed assignment must always be aware of the status of bed availability in the ICU.

Med/Surg Beds

Medical and Surgical beds are required for the majority of patients requiring hospitalization. They come in many different formats and are selected in varying combinations to suit each hospital's needs. Sub-specialty beds are designed for a specific patient type and may be limited to that patient type. Examples are orthopedic beds, cardiac units, respiratory units, stroke units, etc. Other beds are generic and can be used for many types of surgical and medical cases, from appendix and colon resection surgeries to almost any medical type of patient.

Unique cross-functional bed types also exist to serve certain patient populations. OB/GYN beds, for example, serve medical type patients (hyperemesis, vaginal bleeding), patients undergoing surgery (ectopic pregnancy, hysterectomy), obstetric deliveries, and pediatric newborns all in one area.

Pediatric beds tend to vary in type. This is due to the fact that pediatric patients requiring admission to the hospital are often transferred to a children's hospital or a tertiary care center. Hospitals that try to cluster pediatric patients usually find it difficult to maintain an adequate population to optimally utilize the beds resulting in other patient types being placed there. Often, a small pediatric population is simply intermingled within the adult population, which is sub-optimal.

The optimal number of med/surg beds for any hospital is dictated by numerous factors:

- Length of stay for each patient type that will be using the beds
- Volume of complex, longer-term patients. How many cases will stay in the hospital for more than a week? Severe disease processes or wait times for entering long-term care facilities can cause a med/surg bed to be unavailable. How many of these cases does the hospital expect to handle?
- Number and type of specialty procedures such as cardiac Cath, EP studies, specialty surgery, robotics, and transplant centers
- Volume of 30-day readmissions—the more the patients returning to the hospital; the more beds will be needed
- Private or semi-private room availability—A semi-private room is routinely ratcheted down to a private room about 30% of the time because of isolation issues, GI issues, or other factors
- Availability of telemetry systems for patients requiring monitoring

Emergency Department Beds

The volume and types of patients entering the Emergency Department (ED) each day is unpredictable. Hospital rules which prohibit placing patients in sub-optimal areas or managing isolation patients, such as those carrying VRE or MRSA, don't always apply in the ED, especially when it is overcrowded. Patients who might require a private room anywhere else in the hospital are routinely housed in hallways or sit in the waiting room. As discussed above, ED patients are the lowest priority for bed assignment unless they require the ICU, the Cath lab, or have an immediate life-threatening surgical problem requiring the Operating Room. The bed makeup of the ED is therefore varied and includes chairs to handle sheer volume due to space and logistical limitations.

Bed types in the ED fall into several categories.

(1) Trauma beds. These function as the ED's ICU and have a similar priority. Usually the ED is required to keep a trauma bed available at all times.
(2) Standard ED bed. These are med/surg type beds, with similar equipment and resources, such as telemetry, as those on the hospital floors.
(3) Specialty beds. For specialty evaluation such as OB/GYN, ophthalmology, dental, or patients requiring casting.
(4) Outpatient beds/chairs. Patients with minor problems or patients who have been screened and are awaiting test results, etc., wait in available beds and sit in chairs, sometimes in designated areas, and often in hallways when overcrowding occurs.

Basic math often determines how many beds an ED might be equipped with. The average ED patient length of stay is 3 h, which translates to eight patients per bed per day. If an ED evaluates 30,000 cases per year, which is about 80 cases per day, then it would need 10 beds. But this math alone rarely produces the right number and type of ED beds. Several other factors must be considered:

(1) Time of day variability. 70% of ED patients enter during the hours of 12 noon and 12 midnight [37]. This means that 56 of the ED's 80 daily patients crowd in over this period. Over these 12 h, each bed can handle four patients, as each patient cycles through in 3-h segments. So, our 10 beds can only manage 40 of the 56 patients, leaving 16 who cannot be seen in a timely fashion. The ED really needs 14 beds to manage this volume, because patients rarely enter the ED at a steady rate. Then there are the delays that occur for admitted patients. If we now incorporate those patients who will be admitted which is 20% of those 56 patients or 12 patients, we need to factor their LOS in the ED beyond the 3-h evaluation time. The longer that time frame, the less bed availability and the more patients sit in the waiting room awaiting treatment.

(2) Likelihood of delays. An average of 3 h for patient disposition is just that—an average. In practice, this disposition is dependent on multiple extrinsic factors, such as radiology turn-around time, lab turn-around time, specialty consultation availability, drug availability, social work availability, and bed availability if the patient requires hospitalization. If any of these items are unavailable or delayed, the amount of time to disposition the patient will grow, often well beyond 3 h. As that window of time lengthens, with the patient occupying a bed that was calculated to turn over back at the 3-h mark, more and more ED beds are required to maintain patients being seen as they arrive.

Chapter 6

Capacity Management Strategies

A number of strategies surrounding bed capacity management have already been addressed.

(1) Use of Care Management to provide real time reviews of patients for level of care at strategic points within the organization including the ED, Operating Room, and Cath lab.
(2) Centralized Bed Assignment with defined priorities related to bed utilization. Those priorities in order were patients requiring the ICU—then Operating Room and Cath lab—then directs and transfers and finally the Emergency Department.

Here are some additional strategies:

Hospital Prep

In today's healthcare environment, in which many hospitals run extremely high census (over 95% occupancy), it is not uncommon for hospitals to start Monday morning 70 or 80 beds in the hole. Planned surgeries, Cath lab cases, directs,

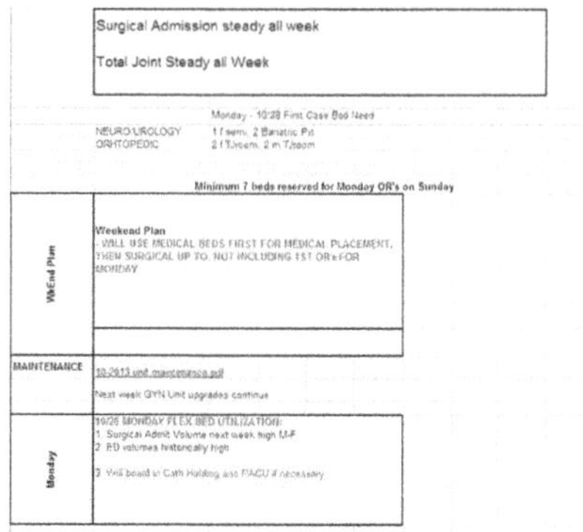

Figure 6.1 Sample of Operational Planning tool for next week volumes (use historical intelligence of Current Week plus next week demand to forecast next week needs).

and transfers, anticipated admissions through the ED and perhaps a quantity of ED boarders might all be waiting for a bed that morning. Many organizations, instead of planning for the inevitable Monday rush (or any other foreseeable bed capacity management issue), start to react only when beds become tight (Figure 6.1).

As noted above, Sunday night, with its lower average volume of incoming patients, presents an opportunity to plan and prepare. During any slower time, it should be possible to prepare the hospital for the inevitable increase in activity. With time to prepare, managers can reserve certain beds, holding them for the post-surgical and post-Cath cases which will begin to flow through on Monday morning. This prevents patients having to be hurried out of these beds and reduces the possibility of a backed up Operating Room or Cath lab. This is also an opportunity to allocate staff appropriately to care for these patients (see Figure 6.2).

It is possible to estimate anticipated volume and plan around it. This type of planning will incorporate:

(1) Scheduled elective surgeries
(2) Cardiac catheterizations and procedures

		Week 27 2013						
		Mon- 28	Tue- 29	Wed - 30	Thur - 31	Fri - 1	Sat- 2	Sun - 3
DOW AVG Jul 2012... Jun 2013	ED ADMITS OBS Service	16	20	18	20	20	21	20
	ED ADMITS MEDICAL-FL	52	70	59	66	54	54	60
	CATH BEDS NEEDED	3	6	6	7	5	1	1
	ED ADMITS ICU	2	3	3	2	2	2	2
	ED ADMITS OR	2	2	3	3	1	1	1
	TRANSFERS/Directs-FL	7	7	7	7	7	3	4
	TOTAL SCHED INPT OR	34	36	26	19	17	2	2
Surgical Schedule	**INPT BED NEEDS**	100	124	104	104	86	63	60
	NEURO/UROL SVC	9	8	3	4	4	0	0
	ORTHO SVC	8	10	5	3	3	0	0
	GEN SURGERY SVC	5	6	8	1	1	0	0
	GYN SVC	3	1	1	2	2	0	0
	VASCULAR SVC	1	2	1	1	1	0	0
	PEDIATRIC	0	0	0	0	0	0	0
	CARDIOTHORACIC	0	1	0	0	0	0	0
	SICU	0	0	0	0	0	0	0
	Surgical Sched Add-ons	8	8	8	8	6	2	2
	SURGICAL BED NEEDS	34	36	26	19	17	2	2

Figure 6.2 Sample of Daily Planning Tool for next week. Uses known fixed schedule plus anticipated unconstrained ED volumes.

(3) Average daily transfers and directs based on prior 6-month statistics

(4) Average daily ED admissions based on prior 6-month statistics

The resulting estimate can help determine staffing needs, provision ancillary services, or prepare to house patients as necessary. This proactive approach, in addition to being more effective, can also be used to help prepare the hospital for the following week's schedule, including the scheduling of surgeries and other procedures. This strategy is most effective if it is centralized, particularly when allocating staff.

In hospitals which are assigning beds to higher priority patients, the ED can get backed up, housing admitted patients who cannot be assigned a bed. An effective means of combating this problem is with staff allocation. Nurses can be reallocated to the ED to provide care to admitted patients, freeing up the ED staff to care for incoming patients. If possible, each population should be kept in a separate area, with admitted patients clustered together. This keeps the extra staff out of the way. I remember suggesting this strategy to a chief nursing officer at a busy hospital. The plan suggested was to hold a number of orthopedic beds Sunday night. This would guarantee their availability for the high volume of orthopedic patients coming in on Monday. The orthopedic nursing staff could then be transferred to the ED to help out with patients boarding there, rather than moving those boarders to the orthopedic unit. The chief nursing officer felt this was unsatisfactory because the nurses from orthopedics would not be comfortable taking care of these patients. The same patients, mind you, who would have been placed on the same orthopedic unit to be cared for under the usual scenario. So, what happened? The beds were held, and the orthopedic nurses were sent home leaving the boarded ED patients to be cared for by the ED nurses.

This demonstrates the disconnect in hospitals on resource utilization and management of the overall system. Another method of attempting to manage excess ED boarders is to place patients in the hallways of the med/surg floors. The idea is that if the staff have to care for a patient in the hallway, they will be more motivated to discharge a patient so the hallway patient will get a bed—Nice theory. In reality, this is difficult to implement. Why? Patient types considered eligible for hallway placement have multiple restrictions. No telemetry, no oxygen, no patient requiring isolation, no patient with gastrointestinal issues, etc. The list goes on and on. I always viewed the placement of patients in hallways as simply removing the crowding problem from the ED to the floors, not fixing it.

Some organizations have designed Rapid Admitting Units (RAU's) to care for these patient types. These units can be expanded or contracted based on need and are staffed predominantly with reallocated staff, who often come from areas in which beds are being prepped for the very patients they are caring for in the ED. This approach is only possible with centralized bed assignment and staffing control. It also requires a broad understanding of the entire organization's needs, beyond any individual area of the hospital.

ED Rounding

A mainstay of proactive hospital management is the practice of daily ED rounding. In the ED, and anywhere else where patients may be housed in unassigned beds, rounding should happen every day. A common time is 7 am. A bed assignment representative, ED charge nurse, and hospitalist or surrogate physician then reviews each patient. This team can determine what type of bed is required (medical, surgical, ICU, Observation, etc.), whether the patient has alternative needs (nursing home placement, specialty equipment, consultation, or requires psychosocial services (homeless, requires medication, requires transfer.

I participated in 7 am daily rounds for over 2 years at a hospital where I'd initiated a morning rounding process. I quickly learned that tackling patient disposition early in the day, every day, can have a huge impact on bed availability. A patient without an acute condition and not really in need of hospitalization might be better served with a transfer to a nursing home, for example. This is better for the patient and frees up the bed for someone more in need of it. But many outside entities, such as nursing homes, can delay patient transfers. In fact, very few nursing homes will take a patient after 4 pm and even fewer will do so on the weekends. Initiating homecare services on a weekend can be nearly impossible and many group home and long-term care facilities actually refuse to take their patients back after a trip to the ED. The morning rounding helped our hospital to identify and resolve these types of issues much faster—which improved levels of care determination and capacity management. Developing a strategy for all those patients who do not need hospitalization has an enormous benefit to the ED and overall hospital capacity management in the long run.

Once each patient's needs are identified, bed assignment can prioritize their placement in a bed. The providers can also now determine where the hospital needs to place emphasis on patient discharge in order to make rooms available. The ED charge nurse can assess daily staffing needs in order to move ED admits out of the ED in a timely fashion.

Effective management of patients awaiting beds is dependent on understanding the hospital's needs as well as the patients. Different areas of the organization may be vying for a limited number of available beds. This is much more important during busy and overbooked weekdays but should be managed every day to institute a standard and reduce variability. Although a mainstay of proactive hospital management, rounding can still become overwhelmed, moving the organization into "surge" capacity management, which we will discuss later.

Chapter 7

Discharging Patients

Getting patients discharged from the hospital is an extremely important component of hospital capacity management. Obviously, the faster patients exit their beds, the more capacity there is for new patients. Once the discharge is ordered, the actual time it takes to execute the discharge is extremely important. Many factors may need to be considered, even from the point of admission. How long is the patient anticipated to be in the hospital? What resources if any will be required at discharge? Are there any issues with medication adherence or acquisition? Will the patient be able to manage at home alone or need assistance? Achieving discharges before noon is also important, providing breathing room for when the incoming volumes start to peak at 1 pm.

It takes a physician or Advanced Practice Professional (APP) to discharge each patient. Surprisingly, this can take more of a provider's time than admitting and rounding put together. In fact, it takes twice as long to discharge a patient, on average, than it does to admit a patient.

Average Provider Processing Times, per patient (not including consulting):

(1) Patient admission 30 min
(2) Patient rounding 15 min
(3) Patient discharge 60 min

There are several reasons for this:

(1) A provider not knowing the patient (it takes time to review the entire medical record)
(2) Issues with setting up follow-up care
(3) Delays instituting home care and other special requirements
(4) Issues setting up drug administration, testing, transport, etc.

These delays are compounded by the fact that doctors consider the discharge process, which is by itself already time-consuming, to be an unpalatable task [31].

It can be put off for numerous reasons:

(1) It is not my patient, so I don't want to make the decision
(2) It is the weekend and I am barely able to see all the patients assigned to me
(3) The patient is too complex, and I just don't have time
(4) The tests I need are not available
(5) I have to do a dictated summary on the patient who's been here for 10 days

Admitting a patient is much more straightforward and less painful. When admitting a patient, it's really about doing three things: examine the patient, write up a history and physical exam, and write a set of admitting orders—done. This is why overnight hospitalist positions are attractive. The clean admitting process is all they deal with, leaving complex and time-consuming discharges to someone else. I remember when

I did some moonlighting as a Hospitalist on the medical floors over the weekend. I arrived to get the list of patients I would need to see and started rounding at 7 am. I found it interesting that none of the private internists seeing their patients or their groups patients arrived until after 9 am Saturday and closer to noon on Sunday, I spoke with a couple charge nurses about the internists' late arrival; their comment was, it does not matter, they don't discharge anyone anyway over the weekend.

A significant amount of discharge difficulty is self-inflicted, however. Providers want set numbers of patients in their assignment list of patients, so that no one physician feels overworked, or they are constricted by residency rules (residents are not allowed to care for more than a certain number of patients at a time), or their patients are strewn about the hospital like grains of sand in the wind.

Each of these realities makes it difficult to manage patient care efficiently under the current dominant model. Without priority rounding, in which providers try to see patients eligible for discharge first, they instead simply start at the top of the hospital and work their way down seeing patients in more or less random order. One hospital referred to their hospitalists rounding as gravity rounding. They start on the top floor and just work their way down. In fact, providers are often unaware a patient may be prepared to be discharged, a fact which causes completely unnecessary delays, and which could be remedied simply with better processes or communication.

There are many more factors in current systems which slow the discharge process, but the key to improvement is to change the dominant care model from scatter-bed, random prioritization, and inefficient rounding to a system which minimizes provider movements around the hospital while maximizing focus and engagement of provider teams on geographically defined groups of patients. This approach is termed geographic staffing.

Geographic Staffing

Most hospitals today have already made some improvements in reducing LOS, when compared to just a few decades ago. One key development has been the introduction of what is known as Hospitalist medicine. As we will see, this approach is a big improvement, not only in lowering LOS, but in delivering quality care. However, the methods of organizing and scheduling Hospitalists can often be greatly improved upon.

Prior to the institution of Hospitalist medicine, patients were cared for by their primary care provider wherever they went within the hospital, even the ICU. A busy primary care physician may have 4 or 5 patients or more in the hospital at any one time. Rounds occurred in the morning before office hours and discharge decisions were made then and there. In the old system, physicians only spent a fraction of their time in the hospital. Decision making, testing and analysis, addressing any unexpected issues, and communicating with friends and family all happened on a far more relaxed schedule than today as a result. There simply was not the same emphasis on rapidly moving patients through the hospital or on being efficient. This was the predominant hospital practice up to the early 1990s.

With the institution of Hospitalist medicine, things have changed significantly. Hospitalists are physicians who are typically trained in general internal medicine, general pediatrics, or family practice, although they may be trained in other disciplines as well. They often are specially trained to manage care for hospitalized patients, as well as to enhance the performance of the institution itself. Their presence in the hospital is far more robust than the old reliance on primary care provider visits. Because they are in-house, and are focused solely on patients within the hospital, hospitalists manage patients more quickly and effectively. This approach has proven to lower lengths of stays, reduce mortality rates, and provide for more standardization of treatment [18].

There are two basic models for Hospitalists Staffing.

The Generic Model

The hospitalist performs all provider functions during their shift—Admit new patients, Round on existing patients, Consult on patients, Discharge patients. Hospital size and patient volume will dictate the number of hospitalists required to manage the daily patient load.

Admit/Rounder Model

The hospitalist performs one of two designated functions. During a shift, each hospitalist either focuses on admitting patients or rounding on patients.

Each model has its strengths and weaknesses. The generic model results in better continuity of care since the provider admitting the patient is also the provider managing the patient. However, it can be very disruptive for a team that is rounding on patients to have to manage an unexpected admission. This approach is quite inefficient in rounding and subsequent discharge. The admit/rounder model allows individuals to go about their day with fewer interruptions. Providers can focus on patients requiring admission or discharge. However, there is less continuity of care, as admitting providers do not provide care for their patients after admission. Both models have intrinsic deficiencies. For example, the majority of admissions actually come between 5 pm and 1 am, which is well after the rounding team has gone home. Both models provide fragmented care.

Many hospitalists are assigned patients and then follow them around, no matter where they may be located within the hospital—just as the primary care provider did before. While

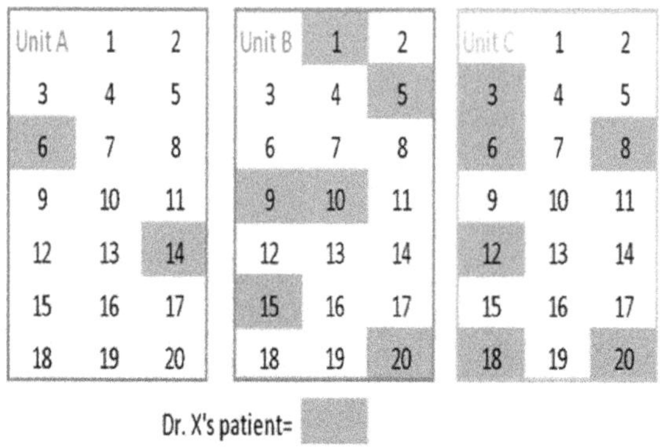

Figure 7.1 Hospitalist Flow where Dr. X's patients are scattered across multiple Medical and Surgical Units.

this is a natural progression from one system to another, it is inefficient. Patients are scattered throughout the system, and Hospitalists must spend a great deal of time moving around in the system just to keep up with their patients. This is extremely time-consuming (Figure 7.1).

This approach also negatively impacts "team-based care" and can impede effective communication with patients, family members, nursing staff, ancillary staff, and sub-specialists. A provider might be assigned six different patients who end up on six different floors of the hospital, greatly impacting their ability to provide for each patient's needs effectively and efficiently.

Geographic staffing is a model designed to address this problem by assigning providers a defined area of the hospital. In its purest form a provider, along with a group of nurses, would actually be assigned a group of rooms and form a geographically stable team. As illustrated in Figure 7.2 with Dr. X and Dr. Y, this arrangement completely eliminates the need to move around the hospital.

There are multiple variations on this theme which can achieve similar improvements in care delivery and metrics. Teams may be composed of only hospitalists or hospitalists

Unit A			
1 RN 1	2 RN 1	3 RN 1	4 RN 1
5 RN 1	6 RN 1	7 RN 2	8 RN 2
9 RN 2	10 RN 2	11 RN 2	12 RN 2
13 RN 3	14 RN 3	15 RN 3	16 RN 3
17 RN 3	18 RN 3	19 RN 4	20 RN 4
21 RN 4	22 RN 4	23 RN 4	24 RN 4

Dr. X=

Dr. Y=

Figure 7.2 Hospitalists are assigned to designated Units with their patients assigned only to those Geographic Units.

and residents or hospitalists and APPs (PAs or NPs) or even a combination of all three (Figure 7.2).

The primary point is to develop teams which stay put geographically and don't roam around the hospital.

A common saying among providers is that the discharge process starts at the point of admission. Geographic staffing is most effective when the admission process works well, ensuring that patients go to the appropriate areas when they enter the system. When a hospital gets this right, it can deliver integrated, patient-focused care throughout the entire patient stay—and that will result in a host of metrics improving.

Observation Units

In recent years, as we have discussed, the population of patients given observation status has become significant. Entering the system primarily through the ED, this group is now a crucial element for capacity management considerations, as well as for hospital structure, bed mix, and staffing.

Most hospitals care for observation patients in the same manner as any other medical admission, using a "scatter-bed" approach, with all its inherent inefficiencies. One reason for this is that observation is viewed as a patient status and little more. The patient's geography (where the patient is physically located) is not considered relevant. But other models exist—and have proven to be superior.

There are four different types of observation units currently in use:

(1) Scatter-bed Unit. The hospital simply places observation patients wherever an inpatient bed is available. Staffing, equipment, testing, and medical needs are considered no different than other inpatients.
(2) Virtual Unit. The hospital simply redefines an existing ED bed as an observation bed. Nothing has changed except the length of stay of the patient in the ED and the utilization of an ED bed for a non-acute ED patient. This approach differs from scatter-bed only by keeping observation patients in the ED rather than on inpatient floors.
(3) Open Defined Unit. Beds are set aside, in a defined location, for observation status patients. Primary Care Physicians, Hospitalists, ED providers, and Sub-specialists may all be managing patients, just as they would in scatter-bed units. The only real difference is a centralized location.
(4) Closed Defined Unit. Beds are designated and centrally located in a separate and distinct area. This unit is managed by a defined staff of observation providers 24/7. These specially trained providers work only in the observation unit, interfacing with hospitalists, primary care physicians, and sub-specialists as needed. This is by far the most efficient type of unit in use today. As such, it will be the focus of our discussion of observation unit design and operation.

Size and Staffing Modeling

Observation patients require a hospital stay, even though they are technically deemed outpatients. During this time, their condition may require additional diagnostic work-up, treatment, serial exams, or sub-specialty consultation prior to further disposition. These patients are often handled in a "scatter-bed" model and are cared for in the same manner as an acute hospital inpatient, causing unnecessarily high costs and multiple inefficiencies. It is possible, however, to analyze a hospital in order to determine the appropriate size of a closed defined observation unit and to properly equip, staff and implement a model appropriate to the hospital's needs.

Unit Requirements Analysis

Over 99% of Observation level of care patients enter through the ED. The volume of patients entering the ED that require a hospital stay can vary depending on the institution and the patient acuity. Currently the average "admission" rate through the Emergency Department is 21% [15]. This is the total percent of patients that are deemed ineligible to go home. These patients fall into numerous categories-ICU, Surgical, Medical, Cardiac, OB/GYN, or Pediatrics. This section deals only with the patients falling into the Adult medical category that are currently viewed as potential observation patients. This volume is usually 25%–30% of the ED patients who require hospitalization. Take, for example, an Emergency Department which treats 50,000 cases per year. 10,500 cases (21%) would require a hospital stay. From 2,625 to 3,150 of these cases (25%–30%) would be classified as observation level of care after an initial review. To determine the number of beds required to manage this volume, the following characteristics of an observation bed need to be taken into account.

It has been well established that the average length of stay of an observation patient is approximately 20 h in an efficiently managed, closed observation unit. The standard scatter-bed approach averages 36 h [16]. An observation bed should be occupied 90% of the time throughout the year. This results in 36 days out of 365 that the bed is empty. If the conversion rate (patient converted from observation to inpatient level of care) is 15% for the bed, the bed holds an admitted patient 49 days out of the year if the bed is only tied up for a 24-h period. If the patient remains longer, bed availability obviously decreases. The result: each observation bed is able to circulate 280 patients per year into discharge status. The total patients handled per bed for the year would be 329. This number adds inpatient conversions (49) to discharged observation patients (280). Since the length of stay for inpatient conversions exceeds the average 20 h by about 18 h, the actual patient per bed usage would be reduced 28 days over the year, from 329 to 301. Now compare that number to scatter-bed, which averages 36-h LOS, managing only 240 patients each year. The closed model produces an increase of 60 patients per bed per year—an enormous capacity boost.

These bed days gained are very significant. The hospital can either use those beds to manage excess volume being cared for in the ED or shrink the organization's footprint by reducing the overall volume of staffed beds required to manage the hospital's patient population. The organization benefits financially while patients benefit from better service, less waiting and more appropriate care (Figure 7.3).

For our 50,000 volume ED, we can calculate that approximately 10 beds would be required (3000 divided by 301) to manage observation volume. The next step is to determine where to put them (Figure 7.4).

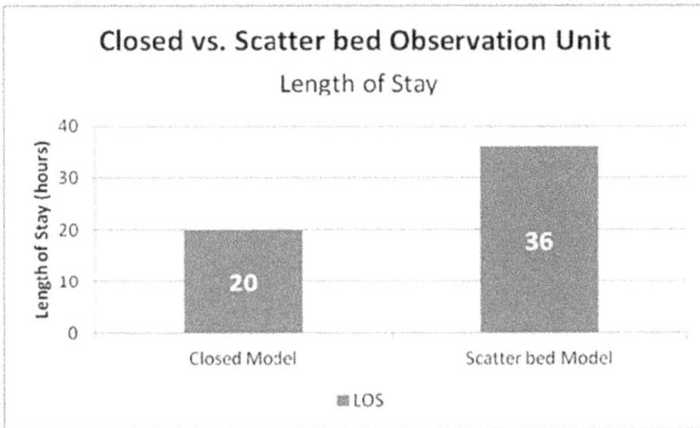

Figure 7.3 Observation LOS in part driven by a "Closed" observation unit / unit geographically located within on location and restricted to "OBS" only patients.

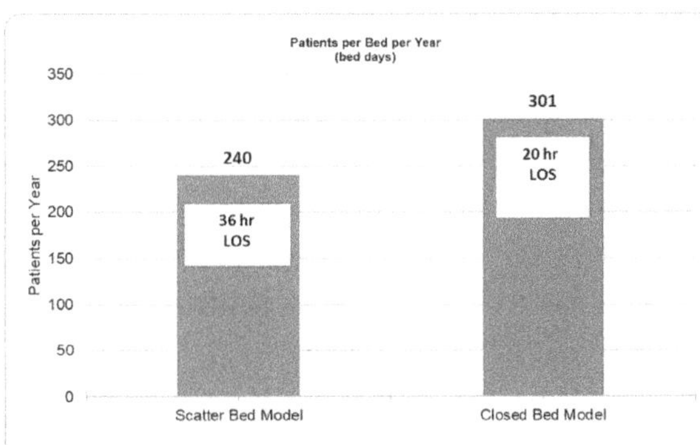

Figure 7.4 Patient numbers and LOS for OBS patients—Closed versus Scattered Models.

Unit Location

Ideally, an Observation unit will be adjoining to or in close proximity to the Emergency Department. This is because:

- The majority of Observation patients arrive from the Emergency Department.
- Close proximity allows for observation providers to see patients quickly for screening purposes.

- Close proximity reduces transport time of observation patients to the observation unit freeing up ED bed capacity.
- Close proximity provides a resource if a patient in the observation unit experiences a life-threatening event requiring emergent intervention.
- Close proximity can assist in the patient's perception of remaining in outpatient status which has consequences for patient education surrounding observation status.

Given the space restrictions within most hospitals, a planned unit may have to be located away from the ED. While not ideal, these units can still be functional, but require the following:

- A well-defined area, with designated beds
- To be equipped and arranged to provide an appropriate environment of care
- To keep observation patients separated from inpatients
- Well-defined staff that are Observation trained and assigned specifically to this unit

Another major factor to consider when planning an observation unit is its staffing. Getting this right is essential to any unit's success. The following is a brief discussion on observation unit staffing.

Staffing

The primary provider in an observation unit is usually an APP (a PA or an NP) working under the guidance and supervision of a physician. 24/7 coverage is necessary in a highly active, rapid turn-over unit. Skill sets, education, training, and experience dictate the volume of patients an APP can successfully manage, but Patient to APP ratios typically range from 12:1 in higher acuity units to 15:1 in lower acuity units. APPs work in 12-h shifts, which work best from 7 am to 7 pm and 7 pm to 7 am.

This staffing pattern is based off a number of attributes. These include, time for sign-outs, patient admission times, patient rounding times, and patient discharge times. When I managed Observation Units, we did a number of time studies that demonstrated on average 3 APP encounters per day per patient. Of these 3 encounters, approximately 2 were billable encounters and 1 was an unbillable encounter. As Observation services have matured, the acuity of patients has increased. What we have observed recently is that higher acuity patients require more frequent unbillable encounters. We found that an unbillable encounter on average consumed 20 min of the APP's time. One can imagine how 5 or 6 additional daily encounters can impact overall unit efficiency. This also has a significant impact on the staffing requirements of a unit. If this is not factored into the overall scheduling, length of stay as well as other operational metrics can be adversely impacted.

When observation units exceed 15 beds, an on-site medical director working independently or in conjunction with the APPs becomes necessary. The unit's physicians usually work day shifts because patients undergo disposition decision making predominantly during those hours. The hours of 7 pm to 7 am are considered to be patient accumulation hours in which patients arrive to the unit, have their History and Physical exam done and their treatment plan initiated by the APP.

Nurse staffing in the observation unit requires standard med/surg floor skill sets. As with APPs, the patient to nurse ratio varies based on patient acuity. Higher acuity units will see 5:1 patient to nurse ratios where lower acuity units can easily manage 6:1. Of note, in the state of California, there is mandatory 4:1 nurse patient ratio for patients requiring telemetry.

Ancillary staff includes Technicians, Secretaries, and Environmental Services. The following ratios for the ancillary staff are based on their responsibilities:

Technician: If doing vital signs, blood draws, patient assistance, etc., the ratio is 8:1.

Secretary: Usually requires 1 individual from 7 am to 11 pm if the unit has fewer than 12 beds. Larger units will require a secretary 24/7.

Environmental services: Usually requires a ratio of 12:1 and one individual in the unit 24/7 to maintain unit cleanliness and room preparedness.

These staffing models may vary from one organization to another and will vary based on the size and complexity of an observation unit. Hospitals that have a relatively small inpatient footprint may not have sufficient volume to institute a defined unit for observation services or even carve out sufficient beds to effectively staff and manage patients 24/7. In those circumstances, an alternative strategy would be to combine other outpatient types that may be clustered with the observation patient population.

These other patient types include:

(1) Extended stay surgical cases or elective post-Cath patients.
(2) Patients requiring certain procedures that require an overnight stay such as renal or liver biopsies.
(3) Patients requiring PICC line placement or other interventional radiological procedures.
(4) Patients requiring chemotherapy infusion that may require 24 h.

These types of patients could effectively be combined with an observation patient population if sufficient training of providers was instituted and the unit had nurses with broad skill sets. Although not a recommended model for hospitals with ample observation patient populations, it is a viable alternative model where appropriate.

Window of Visibility

There is one major factor that results in the failure of many observation units. Termed the "window of visibility," it is the time frame in which the observation unit has empty beds available—for all to see. If we examine the following figure, we can see some striking differences between the ED and the closed Observation unit. Each area runs virtually opposite time frames related to volume and bed availability (Figure 7.5).

As we look at most EDs at 7 am, we find a relatively small volume of patients. The observation unit, however, is at its peak at the same time. As the day progresses and the ED starts getting busier the volume curve starts to rise, but in the

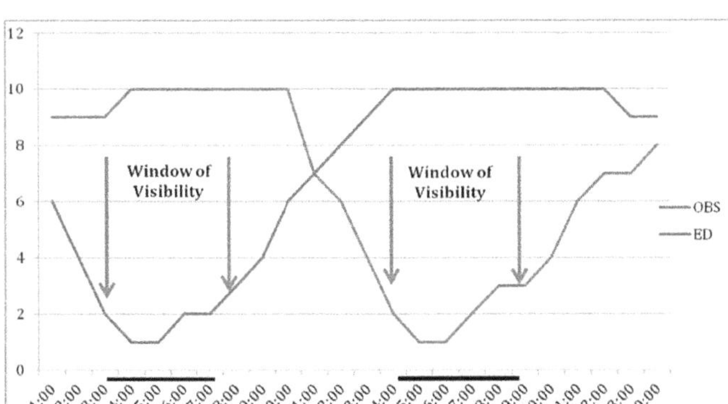

Figure 7.5 Example of the window of visibility.

observation unit the volume curve begins to drop off.
At 2–3 pm, the ED is busting at the seams with patients, the operating rooms and Cath lab are humming and, consequently, room need is at an all-time high.

The one place where beds are visible is the now decompressed observation unit. Suddenly, everyone wants to place other patients in the unit's empty beds. This is the primary failure point for many observation units. Inpatients are placed, they never move, the footprint of the unit contracts and then the observation patients being admitted later that day end up on the floor or remain in the ED with increasing lengths of stay and destroying the efficiency a well-run unit provides. That is the window of visibility.

This inappropriate placement of admitted patients to the observation unit occurs primarily because of reactive management of the hospital beds, a short-term, quick fix, rather than a strategic approach to bed capacity management. This also complicates staffing. Inpatient units that are used to sending nurses home if volume reaches a certain level are used to average LOS's of 3–4 days. Such an approach causes major problems in a high turnover rapid paced observation unit, with a length of stay less than 20 h. Yet, we see this problem occur in many hospitals, causing longer wait times, low patient satisfaction, higher costs, and otherwise negatively affecting multiple areas of the hospital.

Chapter 8

Surgical Short Stay Units

One method of managing this extended stay surgical population is with what we termed a Surgical Short Stay unit. These extended stay surgical patients are not considered inpatients and therefore are not viewed as inpatients under the DRG system. As discussed previously, when a patient is initially being evaluated for a surgical procedure, a series of things have to happen to determine if the patient will be an inpatient or an outpatient.

These patients are divided into a number of different categories.

1. Scheduled Surgical Inpatient
2. Scheduled Surgical Outpatients
3. Unscheduled Surgical Inpatients
4. Unscheduled Surgical Outpatients.

The scheduled patients are then divided into CMS patients or commercially insured patients. To determine which status a patient is placed is based on a number of factors. The CMS patients are placed in inpatient or outpatient status based on a list of procedures and what CMS has determined how that particular procedure will be reimbursed. The outpatient reimbursement is based on an APC (Ambulatory Patient Classification) system. This classification basically determines the government reimbursement for the Physician and the Hospital for a particular outpatient procedure. CMS then provides a window of time on how long the patient can remain in this outpatient status. That window is approximately 6 h. If the patient has no further documented complication from the procedure after the 6-h mark, no further payment is rendered to the hospital. This actually became a serious problem in 2001 when CMS discontinued Observation Care reimbursement because Hospitals were billing for Observation services when patients were placed within the hospital after their procedure for a period of time. Although there is an ability currently to bill Observation care for some of these patients, it's a very small subset. An example would be a patient who has outpatient hand surgery done and then while in the recovery room develops chest pain thought to be cardiac in origin.

So, what is the big deal with these extended surgical cases? Well, it so happens that a percentage of these scheduled outpatient surgeries end up staying in the hospital resulting in higher costs for the hospital and reduced inpatient bed capacity because that bed is being utilized by an outpatient that was supposed to go home after their procedure. Although this does not sound like a significant amount of bed capacity, it can add up quickly. I remember one 500-bed hospital I was at had 8 patients daily being placed into inpatient beds in outpatient status with an average Length of Stay of 30 h per patient. That was 8 patients a day 5, days a week, 52 weeks a year. That was the equivalent of 2,080 bed days. Not a trivial amount of bed capacity or hospital cost.

The concept of managing this population is very similar to the discussion around medical Observation Units. Clustering potential short stay patients of similar types to reduce overall

LOS and therefore costs and improve hospital capacity. One might ask why both patient types are not managed in the same unit?

In theory they could be. There are issues however with skill sets (Need to manage both medical and surgical conditions), patient types (post-surgical patients placed with certain types of medical patients with an infectious process like cellulitis) and perhaps specialty equipment needs. That does not mean that it couldn't be done, it means that those factors would need to be taken into account. One additional factor is based on who is managing the unit and how they are getting reimbursed. For example, if a private group is managing the medical Observation population, they would not be interested in the extended stay surgical population because they wouldn't get reimbursed for care rendered. If providers in the Observation unit are Hospital paid employee's, that might not be a factor. Depending on the hospital volume of extended stay surgical patients, creative management can have an impact on overall hospital capacity by shortening this patient populations LOS.

Chapter 9

Hospital Capacity Management Metrics

As with every other aspect of hospital management, capacity management has its metrics. These are used to determine whether various strategies, processes, and programs are working and typically center on the movement of patients through the health-care system. They not only provide data relating to the hospital's efficiency, but also help to measure how well patients are located and provided for, and in how timely a fashion they are cared for.

Below is an outline of metrics currently being used, it is not comprehensive, but covers how most healthcare organizations are typically being monitored. The list is broken down by different access points to the healthcare system and includes many of the processes which the metrics are tied to.

The Joint Commission, a leading reviewer of healthcare organizations, has determined that patient flow is a primary factor in patient care delivery and patient safety. They have identified a number of patient flow elements for hospitals to measure. In fact, they have made these metrics an important part of their standard hospital review [38].

January 2014—Joint Commission Regulations for Patient Flow in Hospitals.

EP1: The hospital has processes that support the flow of patients throughout the hospital
EP2: The hospital plans for the care of admitted patients who are in temporary bed locations, such as PACU, Emergency Department
EP3: The hospital plans for care to patients placed in Overflow Locations
EP4: Criteria guide decisions to initiate ambulance diversion
EP5: The hospital measures and sets goals for the components of the patient flow process
EP6: The Hospital measures and sets goals for mitigating and managing the boarding of patients who come through the Emergency Department
EP7: Individuals who manage patient flow processes review measurement results to determine that goals were achieved
EP8: Leaders take action to improve patient flow processes when goals are not achieved
EP9: When the hospital determines that is has a population at risk for boarding due to behavioral health emergencies, hospital leaders communicate with behavioral health care providers and/or authorities serving the community to foster coordination of care for this population

While there are many metrics, few rise to the level of importance of length of stay (LOS). It is a primary determinant of hospital efficiency and patient flow and is closely monitored at every institution in the United States. This single metric reflects a hospital's management of discharges, bed availability, artificial and natural variability in patient volume and general efficiency. Higher LOS times are a strong indicator of dysfunction, somewhere within the organization.

Many of these other metrics exist to help pinpoint where these inefficiencies may lie while quantifying their impact. We have already viewed LOS in former chapters and will continue to look at it through the rest of the book.

The following metrics are identified as best practices in various publications [17]. We have included current best-practice measurements for each metric, where available.

Emergency Department Metrics:

Metrics that measure processes

(1) Door to provider time—measured from registration to patient seen by provider—Best Practice < 20 min.
(2) Registration to disposition—Either treat and release, Admission, or Transfer—Best Practice 180 min
(3) Admission to bed assignment—If a bed is available—Best Practice 30 min
(4) Bed assignment to transfer from ED—Best Practice 30 min
(5) Total admission time—Registration to Transfer out of ED—Best Practice 240 min
(6) ED admit to transfer to ICU—Best practice < 60 min
(7) Arrival to EKG time—Best practice < 10 min
(8) Arrival to Cath Lab for STEMI—Best practice < 60 min
(9) Admission to Medication Administration Record (MAR)—Best practice < 60 min
(10) Percent hospitalization request OP/IP ratio—Best practice < 30%

Metrics that measure impact:

(1) Left without Treatment (LWOT)—Patients who enter the ED, are triaged and registered but leave before treatment is instituted or completed—Best practice less than 1%
(2) ED diversion hours—The ED sends arriving ambulances elsewhere due to extreme overcrowding, while walk-in patient wait times become unacceptably long, measured in hours per month—Best Practice Zero

(3) ED boarder hours—These are hours a patient remains in the ED awaiting a bed after the decision to hospitalize the patient has been made—Best Practice 1 h per admission

Emergency Department Ancillaries:

(1) Lab turnaround time—Best practice < 30 min
(2) Plain film turn-around time—Best practice < 1 h
(3) Plain CT turn-around time-60 min

Observation Unit Metrics:

(1) Admit to bed assignment—Best practice < 30 min
(2) Bed assignment to arrival in unit—Best practice < 30 min
(3) Length of stay—Best practice < 20 h
(4) 30-day readmissions—Best practice < 5%
(5) Conversion to inpatient status—Best practice < 15%

Operating Room and Cath Lab Metrics:

There are operating room metrics which look at optimal turnover of rooms, specialty teams, and leveling, among other things, but they are complex and variable. The primary metrics for the Operating Room and Cath Lab regarding patient movement are as follows:

(1) Bed Assignment to Transfer from PACU/Cath Lab—Best practice < 30 min
(2) Percent On-Time starts OR—Best practice > 85%

Hospital Unit Metrics:

(1) Bed assigned to Arrival on Floor—Best practice < 30 min
(2) Discharges before noon—Best Practice > 30%
(3) Room Clean times—Best Practice < 45 min

(4) 30-day readmissions—Best practice < 8%
(5) Complex care patients-patients with LOS > 7 days—Best practice < 2% inpatient volume

These metrics are used by anyone taking a look at operational efficiency. This can include everyone from an ED management company interested in improving its profitability to senior administrators weighing major investments, or government agencies who can levy fines and refuse payments. They matter deeply, not only to the patients who need excellent care, but to the hospital, which needs to maximize revenue and minimize costs. The processes which drive these metrics must be constantly evaluated and improved upon.

The keys to process improvement are the following:

(1) Goal Oriented—Important for the process redesign to be driven by metrics. This way, the success will be measurable and objective. In most process improvement projects, there will be individuals resistant to change and/or cynical of the outcome. When a project is metrics based, it's hard to argue with the numbers.
(2) Involve the people in the process—Those that do the work, know the process the best. If the goal is to design a more efficient discharge process, ask a nurse what they think is essential to the process, talk to the housekeeping staff about how they prioritize rooms to clean, find out what questions the Social Worker has to have answered before the patient leaves. Greater input from those involved will not only create a more streamlined process but will also be conducive to hardwiring the new process down the road.
(3) Simplified, waste free process—When you gather people from each step of the process, they each will likely have suggestions on how it can be improved. By questioning every step of the process and refining what essential

pieces you are left with, the team will come out with a streamlined, highly efficient process. I remember when I was just starting out managing an Emergency Department. We were very busy and had no "Fast-track" to evaluate low acuity patients. My associate director used a video camera to record my progress through the ED with a simple sore throat—total time 120 min. We sat in a conference room with every person who interacted with the patient in the video, getting their feedback on why they did certain things and what they thought should be done. Multiple meetings later and the development of a streamlined process resulted in a fast-track program with a patient LOS of 59 min. It pays to listen and involve everyone.

(4) Standardization—Once the optimal process has been decided upon, the goal is to make sure it happens that same way, every time. Why put the costly time into developing a process if it is only going to be followed when it's convenient or comes to mind? There was a hospital that once got a team together to redesign the care delivery process. The multidisciplinary group designed a more efficient process with standard steps and time frames. Upon implementation of this new process however, the team found that not all disciplines were performing their agreed upon steps in the sequence they had designed. Since their standard process was not happening consistently, and each part of the team could not be counted on, the process failed to achieve the expected results. Standardization has been a key component of Toyota's success in the automotive industry. It is much more challenging to incorporate "Standard Work" in the healthcare arena.

(5) Easily measured—When key players in the process are involved in redesigning their work, a component of their success is developing metrics that are easy to understand

> and measure. In my experience, when someone is crafting a complex metric to measure the success of their project it is usually because they are trying to hide behind the complicated equations used to gauge their success. Much time is wasted in gathering this data, and the creator is rarely satisfied with the result. I have seen that when straightforward numbers are used, leaders take the time to understand how their projects impact the metrics and can speak to how they are calculated. Their depth of knowledge and investment usually result in successful process improvement. I remember in one Hospital, we had just incorporated a new EMR and there were problems with errors in providing transfused blood products to patients. We sat in a meeting to be informed of the new and improved plans to eliminate these errors with the EMR. The presenter then went on to describe a 26-step process to provide a patient a transfusion of blood. We all looked at each other confused since none of us felt we could effectively follow a 26-step process error free.

Understanding these metrics is essential to process improvement. Too many times, organizations attempt to make changes to the wrong area or misunderstand which outcomes need to be addressed. Other projects are too broad in scope, attempting to fix everything with sweeping change. Others are too complex. Many individuals in healthcare like complexity, especially for problems only they fully understand, but this approach is not scalable. It might work in one small area of the hospital—but is doomed to failure outside that individual's zone of control.

Simple, elegant process improvements work the best. They are scalable, such that a process improvement team, tasked with making a difference across the organization, can institute change in one area, then, step-by-step, can roll out a successful pilot program to other units as needed. Keeping things simple reduces the failure rate of an improvement as it is instituted across a variety of departments and greatly improves any implementation's chances of success.

In the next few sections, we will look into several such process improvements, most of which we have seen implemented successfully. Each section begins with a look at the problem area, including key metrics, and then gets into how a hospital could address the issue and improve its metrics—all the while improving the achievement of the ultimate goal, which is to deliver the highest possible level of care and service to patients.

Chapter 10

Complex Care Patients

Not every hospital is able to care for every patient. Acute care hospitals, for example, provide care when a patient presents with an acute medical, surgical, or psychiatric condition. Once the acute condition has been addressed, the patient is relocated if requiring longer-term acute care or specialty care not offered at the current facility. Many complex care patients have more than one issue, making them a challenge to place within the system. An example would be a bariatric, chronic ventilator patient, on hemodialysis with osteomyelitis (an infection of the bone requiring long–term antibiotic therapy).

The challenges surrounding this complex patient population can be daunting. These are patients that many times can't be transferred to any other institution. There can be significant psychosocial challenges, insurance coverage issues, and specialty equipment need. I remember one patient was in the hospital for over 2 years. There were no institutions in the state that cared for ventilator-dependent dialysis patients. The family refused transfer to an out of state facility. So, the patient remained in the hospital proper.

I spoke with a CEO of a hospital who told me of a patient that had a mailbox placed outside their room they had been in the hospital that long. That was unique.

Hospitals employ a number of strategies to manage this complex patient population:

(1) Provide the long-term care delivery within the acute care facility
(2) Transfer the patient to an alternative hospital due to extenuating care delivery circumstances not available at the transferring hospital
(3) Build a long-term acute care facility
(4) Institute agreements with long-term care facilities to accommodate this complex care patient population

Complex Care Patient Types

Respiratory patients:

(a) Chronic ventilator patients
(b) Trach patients
(c) High-flow oxygen requiring patients
(d) Bi-Pap patients
(e) Patients on high frequency respiratory treatment plans—q 1- or 2-h interventions

Nephrology patients:

(a) Hemo-dialysis patients
(b) CAPD patients
(c) Patients with chronic renal insufficiency

Infectious disease patients:

(a) Patients on long-term antibiotic therapy—osteomyelitis, TB, endocarditis
(b) Patients on IV only antibiotic medications
(c) Patients on expensive broad-spectrum antibiotics

(d) Patients on high frequency antibiotic therapy—q 6 h
(e) Patients whose social situation limit the use of long-term IV antibiotics and can include patients with a history of drug use, homeless patients, or patients in care environments that limit treatment options
(f) Patients who are colonized with VRE/MRSA which can make placement in alternative facilities challenging due to private bed needs

Other complex care patient types:

(a) Bariatric patients
(b) Patients with specialty equipment needs—vibrating beds, Clinitron beds, low-air loss beds, and others
(c) Psychiatric patients. These patients are really a combination of the following:
    (1) Group home patients
    (2) Patients with diagnosed psychiatric conditions such as schizophrenia
    (3) Elderly patients with dementia
(d) Patients with Legal guardianship issues
(e) Patients requiring total parenteral nutrition (TPN)
(f) Patients with End of Life issues

Thresholds for length of stay vary from hospital to hospital, but inevitably, complex care patients exceed them. Smaller hospitals that lack sub-specialties such as dialysis, long-term respiratory care, or psychiatric care tend to transfer patients to other hospitals and facilities sooner rather than later. Often, these patients will be transferred to a tertiary care facility with the appropriate capabilities. This dynamic often presents bed capacity management problems for the receiving hospital, which we discuss elsewhere.

Most hospitals have a list of patients that have been in the facility for an extended period. The threshold for placement on the complex care list can vary from a few days to more than a month, depending on the patient's needs and the hospital's policies and capabilities. Every hospital should have a system in place to review these patients. Without a focused approach, these patients are easily ignored. Their disposition can simply be left hanging as their length of stay (LOS) continues to increase. Without focus and a strong process, the hospital may fail to find creative solutions for these patients. Therefore, whatever the hospital's policies, it should assign a team to review each of these patients every day, update their treatment plans, and consider alternative care options.

This team is ideally composed of the following:

(a) Physician leadership
(b) Care management representation from each med/surg/psych unit
(c) Infectious disease representation
(d) Representatives from long-term care facilities
(e) Palliative Care specialist
(f) Administration representative
(g) Home Care Representative
(h) Legal representative

This group should meet weekly to identify those complex care patients who are exceeding defined LOS thresholds and develop treatment plans for each patient. Along with focusing on caring for this challenging group of patients, the team should strive to reduce LOS thresholds and improve patient disposition protocols.

To that end, the physician should engage in frequent rounds, with care management, nursing, and providers to determine where barriers to disposition may exist. The goal of this proactive approach is to provide earlier assistance, such as palliative care, to these patients, many of whom otherwise must wait.

Efficiently identifying and dispositioning complex care patients can have a big impact on bed capacity. Even a small percentage of a hospital's overall patient population with complex care issues can tie up a lot of bed days. 5% of a 300 bed hospital's patients (15 patients) with LOS over 20 days will use up 300 bed days. That is the equivalent of 75 patients with 4-day LOS.

Also important is the fact that much of the high cost of taking care of this population is unlikely ever to be reimbursed. This is because the reimbursement for an inpatient is a Diagnosis-Related Group (DRG) bundled payment. These are based on the patient diagnosis and LOS. Once the LOS exceeds a set time, the hospital no longer gets full reimbursement, making these patients a significant drain on hospital finances.

Chapter 11

Integrated Patient Care

When patient care is a priority, there is a natural integration of more and more elements of their hospital experience, from their entry process through their stay, and finally their discharge. Not only is integrating care delivery service more efficient at delivering care—it's more effective.

An integrated care delivery model starts with the process of admission, then the quick and efficient transfer of the patient, seamless, efficient delivery of care to the patient, and an equally smooth discharge process. The following image demonstrates the key components of this integrated care delivery model.

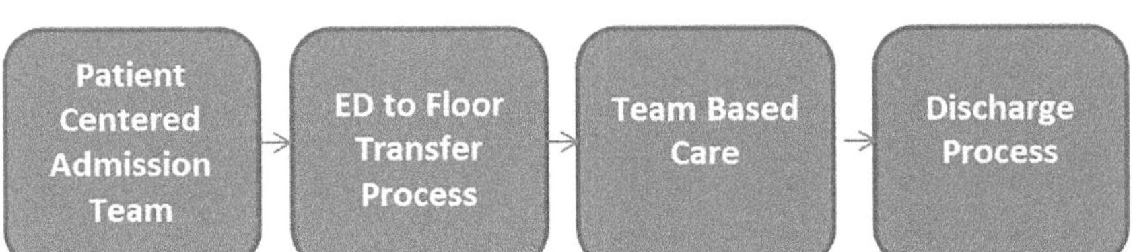

This all sounds very simple. But in reality, it is quite complex, with a multitude of moving parts, departmental handoffs, documents to track, and people to keep informed and engaged.

There are a variety of models in existence, each suited to the size, volume, complexity, and infrastructure of different healthcare institutions. We will walk through a model designed for a large multispecialty organization with very high patient volume. These hospitals often depend on efficient patient processing in order to provide bed capacity. Not every hospital is like this, however. Some very small facilities might find that this particular model is too costly to initiate and maintain.

However, some form of integrated care, for any healthcare organization, can have a huge impact. Rapid admission processing and nursing assessment, error-free patient care and medication delivery, and efficient processes such as medication reconciliation can profoundly reduce LOS, drop readmission rates, and raise patient satisfaction scores. Better managing patient evaluations and assessments also helps reduce costs by enabling more efficient workload rebalancing. If the hospital can better understand patient needs, during more of their stay, it can more accurately assess staffing needs, too.

The Patient Centered Admission Team

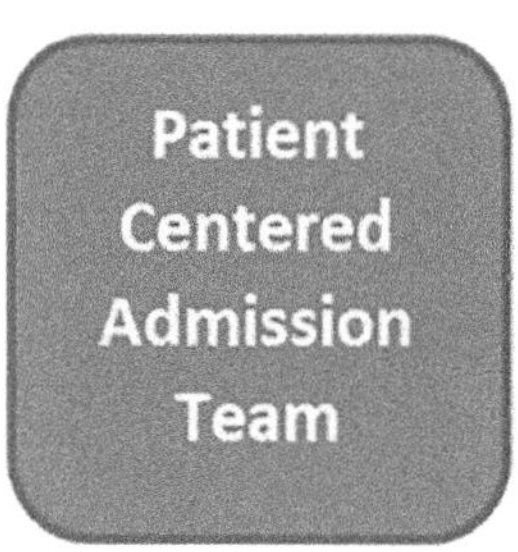

In most hospitals, admissions are processed by a number of different providers acting independently of one another in a sequential order, often resulting in delays, errors, redundancy of effort, higher costs, and lower patient satisfaction.

Sequential processing requires that things be done in a very rigid manner to produce the lowest error rate. A well-known example of this is in the airline industry, where pilots go through a very rigid checklist prior to departure every single time. Healthcare is full of sequential processes, and for good reason, in most cases. An example would be the checklist process prior to surgery, in which, similar to an airline pilot, the surgeon follows a checklist to ensure he has the right patient, the correct surgical procedure on the correct side and so on. I myself recently underwent surgery on my tongue and they actually marked the outside of my left cheek since that was the side the surgery was going to be on. Obviously, I am glad the sequential process helped ensure my surgery was error-free, even though the process took time and resources to complete.

Parallel processing on the other hand is geared for efficiency. Multiple things can be done at the same time. Anyone who takes their car to an oil change shop can see a good example. While one person is taking your information, another is draining the oil and a third is under the hood checking fluid levels. Your car is in and out much faster than if you had changed the oil yourself, in a sequential order of tasks.

There are not many parallel processes used in healthcare because the multiple individuals involved work in separate, siloed environments. Pharmacists have their own process, as do ED nurses, physicians, technicians, and every other healthcare professional. Rarely do they work together in parallel. However, The Patient Centered Admission Team (PCAT) process is a parallel process specifically designed to improve care delivery and efficiency in the healthcare system.

Regardless of admission type and portal of entry, the admission process will typically involve the following providers, each of whom is responsible for a portion of every admission:

Physician—History and physical, orders
Nurse—Nursing Assessment, medication delivery
Pharmacist—Medication reconciliation, medication review, order review, MAR
Technician—Vital sign acquisition, weight, transport set-up, blood draw, EKG

In the majority of hospitals, a patient must wait for each task to be completed, one after the other, and hope that none of the providers or departments involved is having a heavy workload that day. Any delays cause the entire process to be delayed. Before instituting a PCAT, we measured the standard approach to admissions.

The following are actual findings from such a study:

(1) Full history and physical examination (H&P) 25 min
(2) Full admission orders 5 min
(3) Head to toe nursing assessment 60 min
(4) Medication reconciliation 15 min (varies depending on who completes)
(5) Production of an MAR 180 min
(6) Dispense of medications 60 min
(7) Report and handoff to floor nurse 10 min
(8) Report and handoff to floor provider 10 min

Standard Admission Time = 6 h and 5 min

Placing the provider required for admission on a special PCAT team, all of whom are in one place, has a profound effect on performance and patient care. This PCAT team working in parallel and able to coordinate each person involved in the patients care delivery, can immediately provide a complete work-up of the patient. Ongoing care can be provided immediately, with no rework, no error, and no delay. With every component of an admission completed on the spot, the patient is launched smoothly into the system. This approach is quicker, results in fewer errors, improves efficiency, and also boosts patient satisfaction scores.

PCAT Admission Time = 50 min

Patients processed by the PCAT team take on average 50 min from notification to completion of an MAR. This process time includes the exact same tasks as are currently performed by providers to admit a patient.

Some patients, particularly those requiring immediate intervention and disposition, such as STEMIs or unstable surgical patients, will need to be managed wherever their immediate needs land them in the hospital. Other non-ED portals of entry can provide their own highly coordinated teams and processes for streamlining admissions, similar to the PCAT.

The admission process for patients will vary depending on their portal of entry to the hospital.

(1) Elective Surgical admissions are predominantly worked up weeks to months in advance. These comprise the majority of surgical admits.
(2) Direct admissions to the hospital are often similar to elective surgical cases but with a much shorter time frame. They often come, for example, from a Primary Care Provider (PCP) with an H&P and orders written.
(3) Elective Cath Lab patients are handled in the same manner as surgical cases.
(4) Transfer patients are usually managed similar to ED admissions.
(5) ED admissions can average upwards of 45% of all hospital admissions [19]. These patients come in a variety of types:

(a) ICU—these patient's lives are in immediate danger. The ICU therefore requires the highest level of care and the fastest admission and transfer.
(b) Surgical or Cath Lab—also requiring quick admission and transfer, these patients are managed by the surgical or cardiac team. Patient disposition status is determined after the procedure.
(c) Observation—Outpatient status patients requiring a stay in the hospital.
(d) Inpatients—these patients have been reviewed and meet inpatient criteria for a hospital stay.

The volume of admissions per PCAT team is usually 1 per h. The number of teams necessary to process any given ED's patients can easily be calculated. Take for example an ED that admits an average of 30 patients per day, with fluctuations from 20 to 40. To manage 30 patients per day requires 3 teams on 8-h shifts, plus an overlap team for busy periods for a team capacity of 32 patients per 24-h period. Contingency plans must also be considered for those days when volumes exceed this capability.

Concerns are likely to be raised regarding team costs. However, workload rebalancing should result in the teams being fairly cost neutral. Workload rebalancing is simply moving staff assignments to meet needs within the organization. An example of this would be to reduce nursing staff on the hospital floor to reflect a reduction in the need of nursing hours there. Because the PCAT team performs nursing head to toe assessments up front, there is no longer a need for nurses on the hospital floor to perform this hour-long task per patient. A PCAT team that processes 30 nursing assessments a day has removed 30 h of nursing assessment workload from the hospital floor. Reallocating those nursing hours to the PCAT team is more efficient and does not raise costs.

Each member of a PCAT team can similarly be rebalanced. The pharmacist on the PCAT team, for example, significantly reduces intra-pharmacy workloads by performing order entry and MAR tasks up front. This enables a reallocation of pharmacists at no additional cost to the organization—while improving operational efficiency and quality of care.

Physician workload does not significantly change. But the physician's time is spent more efficiently, and he is better positioned to deliver quality care in a timely fashion to his patients.

PCAT Location

In organizations with plenty of empty bed capacity and no delays in bed assignment or transfer of patients from the ED to hospital beds, a roving team should be able to provide the PCAT assessment on the unit. High volume, capacity constricted hospitals, with extended boarder hours in the Emergency Department and delays in patient flow will require an ED-based model. This allows for the process to initiate immediately once the decision to hospitalize an ED patient has been made.

Real-World Impact

In a PCAT system, care delivery begins immediately following the request for hospitalization. This is extremely important in many disease processes that demand ongoing aggressive care. Patients awaiting admission can deteriorate, resulting in longer lengths of stay, increased complications, and increased costs, aside from the obvious increase in danger and discomfort to the patient. Congestive Heart Failure (CHF), Chronic Obstructive Pulimonary Disease (COPD), asthma, dehydration, hyper- or hypoglycemia, and urgent hypertension are just a few examples of conditions requiring speedy admission and immediate care.

PCAT patients also move through the complex hospital system more smoothly and efficiently. They already have a full nursing assessment and their initial medications when they arrive on the hospital floor, which has several key benefits. Floor nurses need not be pulled for extensive periods from other patients, and there is far less chance for medication error. The long wait times for drugs to be delivered are heavily reduced. A recent study, excerpted below with the author's permission, provides excellent data on the impact of a PCAT implementation in practice.

Abstract PCAT: Value of a Decentralized Pharmacist in a Multidisciplinary and Patient-Centered Team in Improving Patient Flow in the Hospital

Patnawon Thung, PharmD (Tables 11.1 and 11.2)

Table 11.1 Primary Impact 1—Reduction in Processing Time from Admission to MAR Completion: 190 Cases

Metric	*Goal*	*PCAT Result Data*
Admit to MAR Time	<60 min	Avg = 49 min
Volume patients/h	1 patient/h	Average 1 patient/h

Table 11.2 Primary Impact 2—Accuracy of Medication—Use of a Pharmacist in Completing Medication Reconciliation at the Time of Admission Results in Significant Interventions and Is Able to Identify Medication List Errors Patients Carry on a Regular Basis. Accuracy of Medication/Reconciliation of Medications at the Time of Admission for 190 Cases over 9 Weeks

Total Weekly Volume Medication Corrections	*Weekly Volume of Medication Edits*	*Weekly Volume of Medication Deletions*	*Weekly Volume of Medication Additions*	*Weekly Volume of Medications Reconciled*
94	16	21	57	420

Table 11.3 Primary Impact 3—Pharmacy Intervention in Drug Information, Drug Interaction, Dosage Adjustments, Pharmacokinetics, Substitutions, and Over Volume of Orders Entered per Week

Weekly Volume Orders Entered	*Therapeutic Substitution*	*Initial Drug Recommendation*	*Drug Pharmacokinetics Intervention*	*Drug Change Occurred*	*Drug Interaction Identified*	*Drug Information Consult*
426	9	2	3	6	1	11

To shed some light on what these numbers really mean, consider just the 94 medication corrections that were made at the time of the PCAT team evaluation. Under standard circumstances, this would have resulted in 94 phone calls being made by the pharmacist to the provider to correct the medication error. That is a lot of provider time if you consider a phone call to be even 1 min, and that every call was answered immediately. That is over 1.5 h correcting medications. Time that could be spent caring for patients. This clearly demonstrates the significant impact a pharmacist can have on medication reconciliation at the time of admission (Table 11.3).

These types of interventions are not only cost effective but profoundly impact patient safety and proper drug utilization. This also demonstrates how workloads are rebalanced. With these orders and interventions now being carried out at the bedside by a pharmacist in real time, the workload of the central pharmacist, who previously performed these tasks in a central pharmacy, is decreased. Moving these tasks to the bedside is clearly safer for the patient, and is more cost-efficient for the hospital, too.

Secondary impacts were found to be significant when comparing PCAT patients to the same patient types admitted by the pre-PCAT methodology (Table 11.4).

Table 11.4 Secondary Impact 1—Length of Stay

190 PCAT Cases	*Baseline Comparison*	*Metric Measured*
3.5 days	5.1 days	Length of Stay

Table 11.5 Secondary Impact 2—30-Day Readmission Reduction

450 PCAT Cases	*Baseline Comparison*	*Metric Measured*
8%	15%	30-Day Readmission Rate

This finding supports the theory that providing care to patients more quickly results in more rapid recovery and an earlier discharge. Patients with many disease processes such as asthma, congestive heart failure, and hyperglycemia require aggressive initial therapy and uninterrupted treatment, even as they move through the system. Patients with co-morbid conditions such as hypertension or diabetes require regular medication, or else they may experience worsening of their untreated co-morbid condition. These types of cases are reflected in this data (Table 11.5).

Simply by performing medication reconciliation up front and instituting more aggressive therapy, there was an expectation that the 30-day readmission for patients treated by the PCAT would be lower than their matched baseline comparisons. The results were astounding. Cutting these readmissions by almost half has an enormous impact on the hospital's reimbursement for services, not to mention patient satisfaction, and, ultimately, patient outcomes.

The PCAT system has a profound impact on organizational efficiency and patient care. There really is no good reason not to do this in every hospital. Also, elements of the PCAT system could be adapted to surgical cases to reduce errors, improve patient management and enhance medication reconciliation—all areas which need improvement.

Efficient Patient Transfer

ED to Floor Transfer Process

Moving patients from one region of the hospital to another is a key component of hospital capacity management—and can impact quality of care. Many hospitals utilize centralized transporter assignment. Requests for transport are placed in a queue and handled in order of priority. This approach is effective when transportation needs are steady and do not vary significantly.

High volume users, such as the ED, with its unpredictable volumes and high rate of admissions to every corner of the hospital, are particularly vulnerable to staff shortages and bottlenecks which can be caused by an overtaxed centralized transfer system. In addition to transporter limitations, bed availability can also become a serious impediment to the timely transfer of patients. This is impacted, as we have discussed, by numerous factors:

(1) Hospital prioritization of patient types
(2) High volumes of ED admissions
(3) High LOS impacting bed availability
(4) Complex care patients in the facility
(5) Transporter staffing
(6) Barrier policies (hospital requirements for transfer)
(7) Lack of defined metrics and accountability
(8) Environmental services staffing
(9) Inefficient bed assignment
(10) Lack of an escalation process

The ED is a high-volume user of transport for its patients; if unavailable, it will run out of beds and completely cease to be able to operate efficiently. Take an ED, for example, that sees 100 patients per day. In a 24-h period, 40 patients will require transport for radiographic studies, 20 will be admitted to the hospital and require transportation out of the ED and 5 more patients will require transfer to a clinic or elsewhere in the hospital. That is a transfer need for 65% of the ED volume every day.

On average, transport time is approximately 20 min. At 65 patients per day, this equates to 21.7 h of time, times 2 for the return trip with equipment and patients. At 1.5 patients per h, this ED will require 43 h of transporter time, equaling 5 transporters per day.

But when we account for ED volume, which is far higher from noon to midnight, we now have to transport 46 of our daily transfers in a 12-h period. This would require almost double the number of transporters.

The hospital queue for transportation suddenly gets backed up, as the operating rooms, hospital floors, ED, ancillary areas, and hospital discharges all compete for overwhelmed transportation staff. Commonly, this results in nurses, care technicians, radiology techs, and even physicians filling in and moving patients. Obviously, this removes care delivery staff from their area, negatively impacting patient care as well as extending the time it takes to move these patients through the system.

The transport process must therefore be designed to adapt to volume shifts while safely and efficiently moving all types of patient throughout the system without delay. As with many other areas of the discussion, transport of patients must adhere to the priority principles of the institution.

Priority 1 Transport

Getting a patient to the ICU in a timely manner can be the difference between life and death. The majority of ICU patients originate in the ED; however, many patients on the floor deteriorate and also require ICU level of care. To get these patients off the floor and into the ICU quickly, many hospitals have developed rapid response teams. However, these teams rarely move ED patients. They focus on patients that are already hospitalized.

The decision to transfer a patient to the ICU can vary from facility to facility. In some places, simple chest pain warrants the transfer, while others require ventilator support or vasopressors before a trip to the ICU is ordered. The less ill the patient must be to be eligible for the ICU, the higher the ICU's use rate will be, and the higher the likelihood that the ICU will be unavailable when it's really needed. Once a decision is made to transfer, then the process of actually getting the patient to the ICU is executed. Below is a breakdown of the process and metrics related to that transfer. As we touched on earlier, a facility should try to keep an ICU bed available at all times. Frequent ICU rounding, bed-ahead plans, specialized facilities for complex care patients, ICU palliative care, and other efforts are all made to keep this vital unit available for incoming transfers.

Some places utilize sub-specialty ICUs, such as CT-ICU (Cardiothoracic) or SICU (Surgical). These can become competitive entities, and organizations in which they exist must be careful to ensure these beds are cross-utilized whenever necessary. With a bed available, the main goal becomes getting the patient there as quickly and safely as possible. Here are the key components for that patient transfer process.

Single Point of Contact

Any process which involves a need to contact multiple individuals or make multiple phone calls will lead to variation, frustration, and failure. This cannot be emphasized enough. I used to tell people, "if you want to establish a process involving the ED and communication, make the process a one number process if you want it to be successful." The key here is a single contact number that connects to a key individual. This person will activate the transfer process. Metrics will measure this point of contact as the start time for the transfer.

On an early trial of a key contact program, we gave a hospitalist a pager and designated them as the key contact for ICU transfers. The pager was an alphanumeric one and received the pages sequentially. The provider answered pages, but in a sequential fashion in which they were received. Because they were receiving pages for other issues as well, our ICU transfer case might not be the first in line to be answered—and this fact caused significant delays.

We they attempted to use a wireless phone but were told by the director of the hospitalist program that the phones did not work above the ground floor. The program, he said, would have to be canceled. We'd been getting some push back about the program, which is often the case when instituting a new process in healthcare and suspected the phone reception wasn't the real issue. The IT folks insisted that the phones worked anywhere in the hospital. Ultimately, I had to get a phone from the ED and ask an ED provider to call me in 5 min. I headed for the hospitalist director's office on the 5th floor. He ushered me in, and we chatted for a bit then suddenly my phone rang. "How about that," I said, "the phones do really work above the ground floor." The program was able to continue, eventually becoming a permanent process improvement program across the entire hospital.

Standardized Response

Everyone understands what is supposed to happen once the key contact is notified. Whatever the organization has determined, their response to be it must be consistent. These ICU type patients usually require ancillary personnel during transportation, such as respiratory therapy if on a ventilator, an RN if on telemetry or have certain drips hanging and perhaps even a physician if the patient may require an intervention in route. This team's arrival time is also measured and evaluated. Processes and functions should be implemented that can enable, facilitate quick response, and result in quicker turnaround times for patients in critical status admission to the ICU. One such process/function developed has been use of:

Early Nursing Intervention Team (ENIT)

The Early Nursing Intervention Team (ENIT) is an evidence-based concept, which was developed in hospitals by teams of nurses including ICU and General Care Unit staff nurses as well as clinical nurse specialists. This works when supported by Nursing and Provider Leadership.
The goal of ENIT is to improve patient outcomes by providing early response to patient deterioration who require critical care.

ENIT is a nurse-to-nurse consultative program which provides support to novice clinicians by clinical experts.

The ENIT Responder is the ICU Charge Nurse, who does not carry responsibility for a patient assignment in the ICU. Rather than only respond to calls for assistance, as a typical rapid response team would, the ENIT Responder proactively rounds twice daily on the general care units.
The rounds encourage communication, provide a forum to address staff questions and concerns, and identify patients that concern the staff on the general care units.

Additionally, staff nurses are encouraged to consult with the ENIT Responder for any patient care questions or concerns they may have at any time. In addition to rounding and providing consultation to the staff on the general care units, the ENIT Responder attends any Code Blue (cardiac arrest) or STAT page on the general units and facilitates patient transfer to the ICU if necessary. Establishing ENIT requires the approval and recruitment of additional resources for the ICU as well as the general care units. These additional resources ensure that as the ENIT Responder, the ICU charge nurse does not have an assignment within the unit and is therefore available to the general care unit staff.

ENIT, where used, has resulted in improved communication and collaboration between the ICU nurses and general care unit nurses. ENIT nurtures and guides the novice general care unit nurse in developing assessment skills and intervening appropriately in complex patient care situations. Utilizing Situation, Background, Assessment, and Recommendation (SBAR) processes, ENIT has standardized communication, providing a definitive approach in communicating between nurses and physicians [40].

Bed Assignment

The third element of transfer is often forgotten. In a centralized bed assignment system, the bed the patient is being transferred to must be assigned by someone. An important reason for this is that patients in the electronic world can in many instances not get the treatment required once transferred, if they are not electronically placed in the bed they have been assigned. Nursing documentation and the ability to provide medications out of an electronic medication dispensing system may delay therapy. Thus, the need for bed assignment and the last key metric that requires measurement

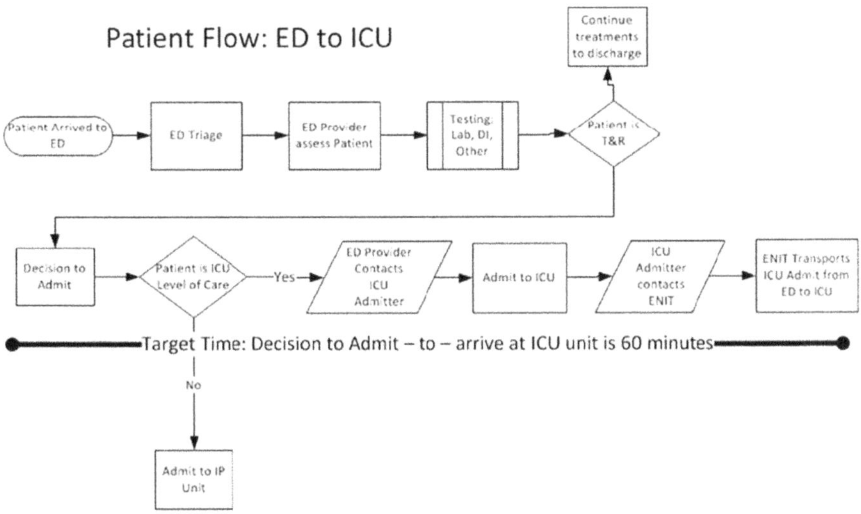

Figure 11.1 ED to ICU flow.

in this process: arrival time in the ICU bed. The entire process forms the final stage of a larger process which begins with the patient's arrival in the ED and ends with arrival in the ICU, and is expected to take no more than 60 minutes after the ED's decision to place the patient in the ICU (Figure 11.1).

Priority 2 Transport

The transport of a patient out of the PACU has important implications. The PACU has limited bed availability and requires a flow of patients out of the area to prevent operating rooms backing up and becoming non-functional. This becomes extremely expensive, not only in terms of delivery of care to patients, but, at $1,000 an hour to run an OR room in financial terms as well. Good capacity management, such as holding beds overnight for known volumes of cases, in conjunction with efficient transportation, can make getting patients out of the PACU very streamlined and efficient.

Because patients can have their bed assigned prior to their surgery, delays should be minimal. A transport time of 30 min out of the PACU or Cath LAB is very achievable (Figures 11.2 and 11.3).

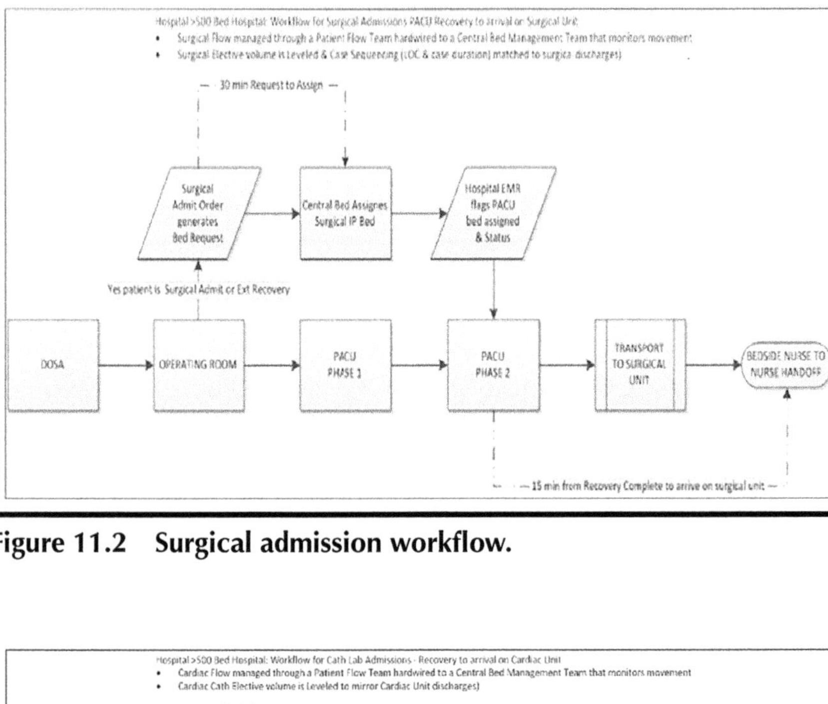

Figure 11.2 Surgical admission workflow.

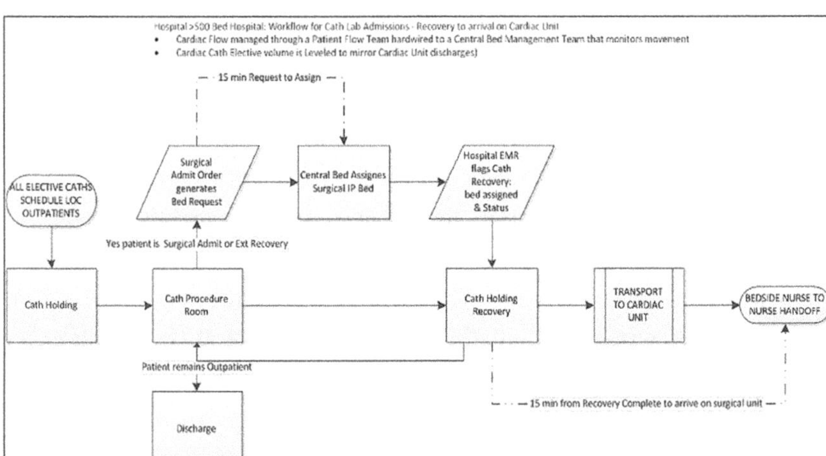

Figure 11.3 Cath lab admission workflow.

Priority 3 Transport

ED to Hospital bed—this would be the same for observation, floor, even a surgical case like a post-appendectomy would apply. This transport process is dependent on a number of interactive elements working together. Bed-assignment metrics need to be closely monitored, providing communication of patient type and bed need as early as possible, then assigning the correct bed type (if available) within 30 min. Transport is then engaged, along with properly trained personnel.

Telemetry, which is necessary for certain cases, is often overused, causing a major barrier to transportation efficiency. A hospital I once evaluated was sending everyone to the floor on telemetry, even cellulitis or kidney stone patients. This overuse of telemetry was not only costly from an equipment perspective; it was costing them almost 2 Full-Time Equivalents (FTEs) of RNs just to do the transport. Shortages of portable telemetry equipment were causing additional delays, as were wait times for available RNs who were required to travel with telemetry. Few patients outside those admitted to the ICU require telemetry monitoring unless the patient is on specific cardiac medication drips (Figure 11.4).

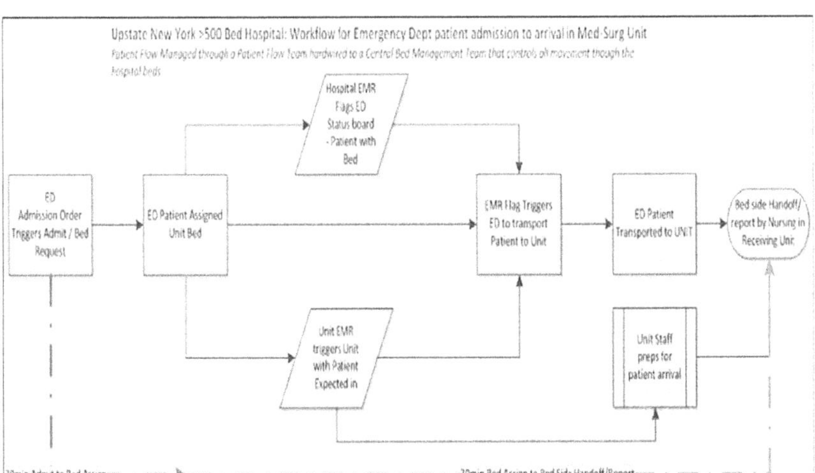

Figure 11.4 Emergency Department patient workflow.

Team-Based Care

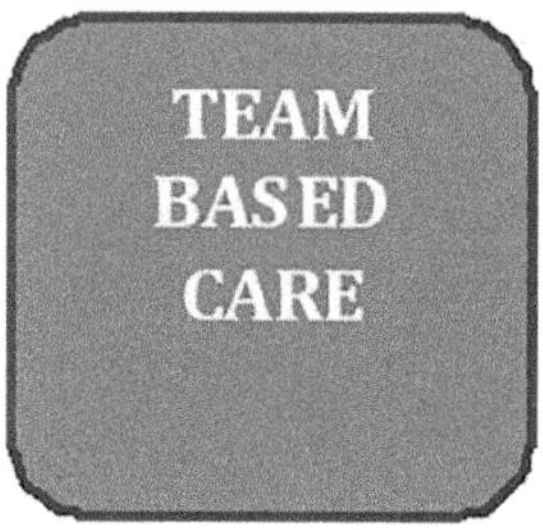

Years ago, before the electronic revolution, I was a resident in internal medicine. We carried a fairly large patient population (20 patients) that was scattered throughout the hospital. Our day would start at 6 am in a large room with sign-outs on any patient who experienced a problem overnight. Then we were off and rounding on patients with a cart full of charts that would acquire orders during rounding, then left off at the secretary's desk for transcribing. Rounding would be followed by a trip to the lab to get patient lab results, then microbiology, then radiology to review x-rays, then back to the floors to check on patients who had any abnormalities that needed to be addressed while fielding calls from the ED for new patient admissions that needed to be seen. I wore a pedometer one day while an intern and logged 8 miles of walking. Clearly, not very efficient.

The advent of the electronic age changed all that. We can acquire and distribute information more efficiently. Electronic Medical Records (EMRs) can provide at a glance each patient's vital signs, labs, medications, radiographs, special study results, and a consult note, while enabling the writing of orders, discharge instruction information, and prescriptions. This has saved providers countless hours of time and many miles of walking around in circles. However, the process of providing care in a fragmented, scatter-bed designed delivery system has remained, retaining a great deal of the inefficiency of the past.

There are organizations that have attempted to change this way of doing things, with some success, but by and large the process of assignment and rounding remains largely unchanged. Doctors and staff, alas, still must walk around in circles.

Over the years, I have heard many excuses for this. Perhaps the most popular defense of the scatter-bed system is continuity of care. This rationale dates back to the days of Primary Care Physicians (PCPs) caring for their patients in the hospital. With so many PCPs rounding, no other system made sense. Continuity of care meant the same PCP would care for his patients from the ED to discharge. But today, all those PCPs have been replaced by the hospitalists who work in the hospital.

It is not unusual for a patient to be seen by many providers during their stay. Here's a typical scenario: Patient enters the ED Friday at 5 pm and sees ED provider 1, who starts a work-up, but signs out to ED provider 2, who determines need for admission at 10 pm. The patient is then seen by provider 3, a Hospitalist, who writes up the admission and the patient is transferred to the floor. The next day the patient is seen by provider 4, another Hospitalist, and his team. This provider goes off service the next day. The patient is then picked up by Hospitalist provider 5. The continuity of care which was provided by PCPs no longer exists.

Equity of work is often raised as a barrier to replacing scatter-bed systems. Many programs use work equity to maintain specific team sizes or admission volumes without necessary regard to patient placement. This only exacerbates the problem of scatter-bed fragmented care delivery and is a good example of how hospital priorities skew to provider needs rather than those of the patients.

Another issue raised in resistance to reform is a hospital's residency program. The residents need to see the patients, of course. But if scatter-bed were replaced with some geographically based system, the way we integrate residents might need to be adapted too. While I see this type of resistance as no more than a minor issue, it is sometimes posited as an iron-clad argument for keeping things the way they are.

Finally, fears that providers would become bored are raised. Seeing the same type of patients in the same specific location might prove too boring and providers will stop enjoying their jobs and become demoralized. This argument is predominantly used when specific patient types, like observation patients, are clustered together.

Excuses aside, the bottom line is that scatter-bed systems, and the workflows they necessitate, are inefficient. This inefficiency has far-reaching effects and consequences throughout the entire hospital and its patient population. If we truly focus on patient care and stop worrying about whether providers will get bored, we can accept that the system simply needs to change. This shift revolves around geography and staffing models. What is referred to as geographic staffing and team-based care delivery models.

We must also understand that a shift to geographic models, with team-based care, will require a cultural shift within the hospital community, as well as changes in behavior.
It requires standard work, is time sensitive, and requires active communication with nursing, patients, family, and others.
The new system will require staff to remain in the geographic area during their entire shift and, they must be accessible.
These are difficult and dramatic changes in the behavior of highly intelligent, independently functioning individuals, called doctors. Nurses, it should be noted, have already mastered geographic staffing and from my experience are very receptive to assisting in team-based models.

Team-based care is an organizational model that completes the long transition from PCPs caring for patients scattered throughout the hospital to a far more efficient, patient-centered system using hospitalists, geographic staffing, and standard work practices. Team-based care has proven highly successful in practice, leaving very little doubt that all those excuses for keeping things the way they've been for nearly a century are just that—excuses. There are variations on the central concepts, of course, but we will look at a typical 12 room model (A Module)—one that has been successfully implemented and is running well in hospitals today.

The care delivery team for this 12-room model consists of a physician, two RNs, and two technicians. The physician will care for 12 patients, while their RNs and technicians will each care for 6 patients. These team members, working in the same area of the hospital, provide the majority of both care delivery and decision-making surrounding the patients in that well-defined area. Additional ancillary team members are also essential to the efficient delivery of care to these patients. These ancillary team members can cover a greater number of patients. In our model, each will be responsible for 24 patients, except for environmental services, with 12 each. These team members are a care manager, a social worker, a secretary, a pharmacist, and two environmental service workers.

Working together, each team member becomes an active participant in the needs of each patient and can provide valuable input regarding their care. Twice a day, the entire team huddles together for approximately 5–10 min. Any patient status changes or changes in care plans are shared, keeping everyone informed and current. In the huddle, everyone reviews the entire patient census, and can determine changes in treatment, challenges to discharge, and proactive opportunities to intervene with patients or communicate with family members. In this way, essential communication is effective, consistent, and highly efficient. Example of a two-team-based model is shown in Figure 11.5.

Unit A			
1 RN 1	2 RN 1	3 RN 1	4 RN 1
5 RN 1	6 RN 1	7 RN 2	8 RN 2
9 RN 2	10 RN 2	11 RN 2	12 RN 2
13 RN 3	14 RN 3	15 RN 3	16 RN 3
17 RN 3	18 RN 3	19 RN 4	20 RN 4
21 RN 4	22 RN 4	23 RN 4	24 RN 4

Dr. X=

Dr. Y=

Figure 11.5 Example of a two-team-based model.

Standard Work

This process of standard interaction between primary and ancillary team members follows what is termed "standard work." Each team functions in the same manner each day without variation unless something serious disrupts the team's standard work, such as a patient becoming unstable or requiring an eminent higher level of care like the ICU. Interaction of team members at sign-outs is extremely beneficial.

This book contains a lot of discussion of standard work. In many ways, it is the way we all live our lives. A good example of this is that when I get up in the morning, I have a set routine:

Step-1 shower
Step-2 shave
Step-3 dress

Step-4 prepare breakfast
Step-5 eat breakfast

Now if I decided that tomorrow I would change up and eat first, then shave then shower, etc. and then the next day pick a different routine, I would probably drive myself and my significant other crazy. But this is exactly what we do in healthcare when provider A and provider B, each have their own way of doing things and try to coordinate care delivery for the same patient. Care delivery becomes chaotic and many times mistakes are made.

Simple as this may seem, providers resist whenever standard work for care delivery is discussed. Some have suggested that their creativity might be stifled or that we are trying to get them to practice "cookbook medicine." However, recent studies have demonstrated that medication errors occur in 5% of hospitalized patients while major errors such as wrong-sided surgeries continue to occur throughout the healthcare system [31]. These types of errors are often caused by non-standard processes and could be greatly diminished, as they have been in many other industries, by using standard work practices.

I doubt seriously that Toyota deviates from standard work when assembling cars. While there will always be a need for creativity, problem-solving, and quick-thinking among providers, our system would benefit a great deal from standard work in care delivery.

An Example of Team-Based Care Staffing

When nursing staff sign out at 7 am, the physician should be an active part of that sign out to determine any issues which may have arisen overnight. The nurses also are very adept at knowing who may well be ready for discharge that day or what barriers to discharge have been identified. Examples

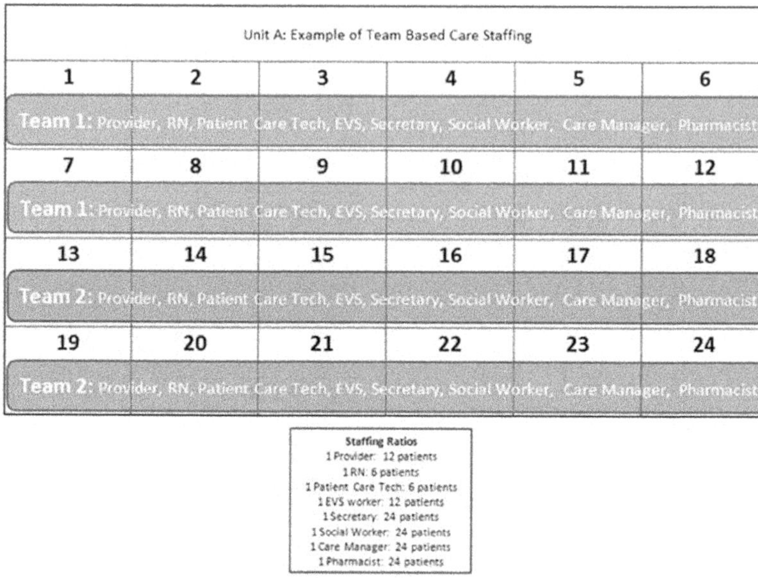

Figure 11.6 Example of team-based care staff pattern.

would be a change in the patient's vital signs, evidence of a fever, pain, nausea or vomiting, or numerous other possibilities. I remember when we attempted a pilot of team-based care on a hospital unit and requested the physician be on the unit at 7 am to listen to report with the oncoming nurses on their team. We were told in no uncertain terms after 2 days; the nurses didn't provide any valuable information and there was no reason to continue joining them in sign-outs (Figure 11.6).

This is another example of the marked difficulty in attempting changes in physician behavior. The following is an example of scheduled standard work for a modular team. The purpose of team-based care is to reduce the redundancy of work, eliminate variations in communication to patients regarding their status, efficient work-up, and disposition of patients and eliminate the significant waste of provider time spent traveling around the hospital. Concentrating the team in a closed unit area significantly reduces time spent on phone calls, shrinks wait times, and improves communication with the patient, family, and sub-specialists. Well-defined standard work practices make any movements between "Modules" seamless, regardless of patient type.

Another benefit of the team-based modular system is the ease of quality tracking and comparisons. Falls, hospital acquired infections, core measures, readmission rates, length of stay, patient satisfaction, and many other items can be evaluated for each module. This helps to identify and contain any problem areas which might arise, and to institute and standardize practices which are proven effective (Figure 11.7).

The modules that function best can be examined more closely for specific processes and procedures, which can be identified as best practices and instituted throughout the institution.

Although team-based care is focused on the medical patient population, it by no means is limited to that group. As medicine evolves over time, procedure-based specialties will no longer provide primary care for hospitalized patients. Specialties such as Neurosurgery, orthopedics, cardio-thoracic, and others will perform the procedure and then allow alternative providers (hospitalists) to manage the patients stay in the hospital. High acuity facilities with many specialties have constructed their hospital in segregated areas specific to a patient's needs. This may be secondary to equipment (bariatrics' for example) or may be secondary to ancillary personnel (orthopedics and the use of physical therapy for example, Figure 11.8).

The design of the modular, team-based care model could easily be adapted to any specialty. However, the success of modular, team-based care is limited, if other components of the organization function inefficiently or have different priorities. The other components are as follows.

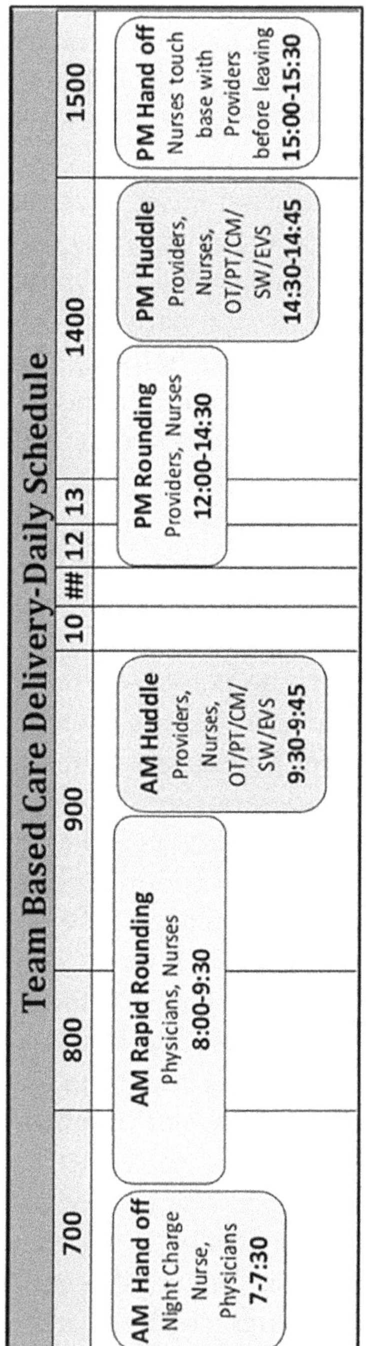

Figure 11.7 Team-based care daily work timeline.

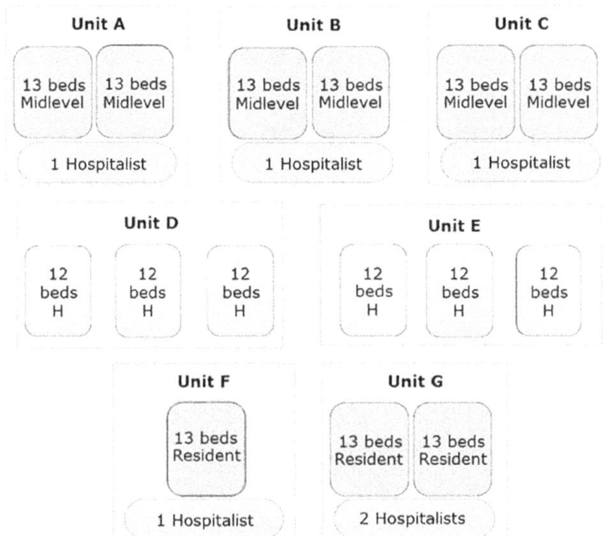

Figure 11.8 Team-based care unit structure.

Testing

Approximately 70%–75% of patient evaluations are completed in the ED. Additional testing, however, can be a significant source of delay in patient disposition. MRI, ECHO, Stress Testing, USN, CT scans, etc. can all be rate limiting steps in the completion of a patient's evaluation. Often, a hospital facility performs studies for both hospitalized patients and outpatients, and finds itself giving priority to scheduled outpatients, causing everyone else to wait. This may be due to several reasons: reimbursement, control of a scheduled population, and easier testing are chief culprits. When this occurs, the hospitalized patient is processed later, delaying the decision-making process, which delays consult acquisition and ultimately is reflected in an increased LOS as a result.

Every department needs to work closely with the hospital to make sure hospitalized patients are prioritized for testing. The team-based care provider must be able to communicate to the testing department what priority should be given. Obviously, a life-threatening test takes absolute priority but after this comes "the day of discharge-dependent testing," tests whose results will allow a disposition decision to be made, especially if the disposition decision is discharge.

Day of Discharge-Dependent testing is an important component of the team-based care model. It should also be well established throughout the hospital community that not every test has to be top priority. Many tests can be accomplished on an outpatient basis, for example, and need not bump a discharge decision on the priority list. The more everyone understands this and communicates as a team, the better the entire system will work.

In January of 2020, CMS instituted a mandated appropriate use imaging program. This program will require physicians ordering expensive testing on outpatients to get prior approval for the test. The use of an algorithm to determine appropriateness of the test will be required. Starting in 2021, if a physician fails to do this, the test will not be paid for by CMS [39].

Consults

Similar to testing, consultation should also be prioritized. Obviously, an emergent consult such as a patient suffering an MI requires the immediate attention of cardiology, but patients whose discharge is dependent on a consultant's recommendation are high priority, too. If consultants simply take patients to be seen in the order given without any idea of priority, patients whose discharge may have been implemented that day will stay in the hospital an additional day. So, Discharge-Dependent Consultation is a key component to efficient team-based care. Proper use of consults is also important, since, like testing, many consultations could be outpatient-based.

Pharmacy

The role of pharmacy in the team-based care model is to assist in determining issues with drug interactions, optimal drug utilization, cost effective drug use, proper dosing, and non-formulary substitutions. They can also be of considerable assistance with patients who wish to take their own medications.

Pharmacists also have a role in unit huddles to be updated on patient discharges. Teaching patients about their medications has become a significant component of the discharge process, resulting in reduced readmissions where it is done well.

Environmental Services

The primary role of environmental services is to keep the unit clean and turn rooms around when patients are discharged. They are a key component in the efficiency of a team-based model. They should be active participants in the huddles to determine which patients are likely to go home that day.

Most discharges do not begin until 10 am and then end by 9 pm at night. By 10 pm, all discharges and bed cleans should be completed unless a patient is transferred for some reason. I remember one episode when I was a member of a patient flow committee and the Director of Environmental services was scheduled to give a presentation. The Director had decided that rather than use one environmental service person to clean a room, they would use two. This would result in the room being cleaned in 20 min instead of the usual 30. Now I listened to this and thought it somewhat strange. A normal room clean takes 30 min or 2 rooms per h. So, during an 8-h shift, an environmental cleaner should be able to clean 16 rooms (2 × 8 h). If now the plan was to use 2 cleaners to clean a room, the cleaning pair would be able to clean 3 rooms per h or a total of 24 rooms (3 × 8 h). However, if I'm using 2 independent cleaners able to each clean 16 rooms in 8 h, that's a total of 32 rooms (2 × 16). With this new plan there would be a room cleaning bandwidth loss of 8 rooms. When this factoid was pointed out, the new plan was shelved.

Technicians

These individuals provide assistance with vital signs, blood draws, patient personal hygiene, feeding, ambulating patients, and multiple other tasks. In the team-based care model of 12 rooms, there should be at least one, but preferably two technicians. A key component of the tech's responsibilities would be the assistance in the discharge process and the admission process. This sped the process of moving patients in and out of the facility as they are discharged and admitted.

If we examine the team-based care model in more detail, the impact can be better understood. The following standard work is based on the modular care model previously discussed.

Seven Standards of Team-Based Care

1. Geographic Staffing. Having care providers all in one location allows for timely and efficient communication between physicians, nurses, care managers, pharmacists, and other team members. Patients assigned to the team are also located in the immediate area, eliminating rounding inefficiencies and optimizing staff time spent on patient care.
2. Morning Sign Out. Physicians are able to participate in the handoff between the night nurse and the day nurse to learn of any issues that happened overnight that may adjust their priorities for the day.

3. Morning Rapid Rounding. Multidisciplinary team rounds on each patient and discusses the plan for that day. Spending about 3–5 min with each patient as a unified team allows for thorough communication about the needs of the patient. Using a simple stopwatch has been shown to keep the team on track.
4. Morning Huddle. Multidisciplinary huddle to review every patient on the unit. In addition to updates on patient needs, this is an opportunity for everyone to discuss potential discharges or discharge issues for the day.
5. Afternoon Rapid Rounding. Multidisciplinary team rounds on each patient to check in on any testing results and plan for the evening.
6. Afternoon Huddle. Review today's discharge status and discuss any issues. Prepare for tomorrow's discharges.
7. Afternoon Sign Out. Physician check-in with nurses before leaving to review patient's needs for the evening. Any special orders can be reviewed.

When in place, modular team-based care, using a geographic staffing model, will have a significant impact on the hospital's overall performance. In practice, we have seen this model consistently improve key metrics such as the following.

Length of stay. Improvements in communication among care providers, combined with focused, efficient care delivery has shown to reduce LOS.

Readmission rate. All-important 30-day readmission rates drop significantly. Better patient education, standard work hand-offs, consistent communication, and focused care keep patients from having to come back to the hospital once discharged.

Patient satisfaction. Directly affecting reimbursements under the ACA, this crucial metric has been shown to improve under team-based geographic models. This is most likely due to the effective, timely, and consistent communication by providers and nurses and has a direct effect on hospital reimbursements.

In our experience, working in many hospitals over the years, and consulting with many more, we have found that the degree to which team-based care and geographic staffing models achieve positive impact is limited only to the quality and success of implementation. When done well, the impact we have seen, and documented, is truly game-changing [32]. As with any program implementation, it does less well when implemented with half-measures and heavy compromises [20].

The danger here is that some administrations may attempt to "try" this much-discussed new model, but not truly commit to it. Then, having proven it flawed, they can dismiss it and return to the old scatter-bed system, which, as we discussed above, many in the healthcare system seem to prefer.

Standardized Discharge Process

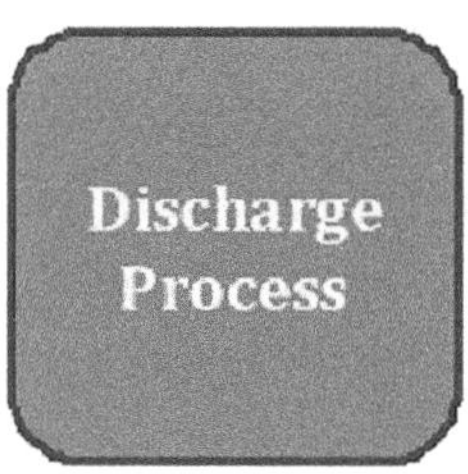

The final stage of the integrated care delivery model can be extremely complex. While some patients are sent home, many are discharged to rehab facilities, nursing homes, hospice, and a variety of other places, each with its own set of problems and requirements. As noted above, the process of discharge should really start at the point of admission. Getting the patient's medication reconciliation done correctly at the point of admission is extremely important.

Discharge Definition. The patient has left the bed and the bed has been cleaned and notification has reached bed assignment. The reason for defining discharge is that various individuals have a different definition.

For example,

Provider definition—When the order is written (many times providers skew this number by writing discharge-dependent orders) This can in reality add hours to a patient's discharge and gives bed assignment a false sense of bed availability. When consulting, a question, I would routinely ask Hospitalists would be "What percent of discharges before noon do you have?" The answer would usually be something like this. "Well, the order is written 50% of the time." When I would ask bed assignment it would be <10%. Simply writing an order without that order being communicated can result in significant delays. Another caveat is the writing of "discharge-dependent orders." This looks like the discharge order was written timely but is dependent on a consultant or a test being completed. This results in gaming the system, not improving it.

Nurse definition—When the patient has received their discharge instructions

Transport definition—When they take the patient to the discharge area

Environmental service definition—when the room is clean

Bed assignment definition—When the bed is ready for the next patient

Communication is probably the biggest factor impacting quality and timeliness of discharge. Patients, family members, or friends need to understand and be aware of a pending discharge as soon as possible because home care delivery, transportation issues, medication issues, and follow-up needs can impact the patient's well-being. By addressing these factors early in the patients stay, frustration and discontent can be avoided. Furthermore, we have seen that a standardized discharge process can help reduce readmission rates; an impact which is positive for patients and the hospital [33].

The following is a standard practice which should be followed on any patient admitted to a hospital unit and can easily be checklist-based.

(1) Anticipated discharge location—home, nursing home, rehab, etc.
(2) Transportation needs—family, friends, taxi, stretcher, etc.
(3) Medication needs—insurance, available financial resources, etc.
(4) Anticipated home needs—equipment, oxygen, PT, home care
(5) Patient follow-up needs—PCP availability, sub-specialty needs, etc.

Addressing these five questions at the time of admission will provide team-based care member's insight and a head start when focusing on discharge issues for their patients. These components are the starting point. At the time of discharge, additional information will be required, as will a strategy for making each patient's discharge a success. There are several considerations and strategies that will need to be considered.

Disease education. Patients who leave the hospital without properly understanding their health issues often return, sometimes even sicker than when they first arrived. It is crucial, both for their health, and today for the hospital's reimbursements, to ensure each patient understands their own condition and care requirements. Achieving this often involves multiple team members. For example, a newly uninsured diabetic without a PCP will need diabetic teaching, medication, dietary instruction, and a follow-up physician. This patient will require input from a nurse, physician, social worker, pharmacist, and a diabetic teacher before discharge. Skipping any of these could cause this patient to get sicker and return to the hospital. I remember one hospital I was working at did not have a diabetic educator on the weekends. Many times, patients would sit all weekend until the educator arrived on Monday to set up resources, provide instruction on how to use equipment, etc. To allow these patients the ability to be discharged on the weekend, we set up a unit nurse educator position with the weekend staff, placed a pack of diabetic teaching material and equipment in the electronic medication dispenser and now had the ability to discharge on the weekend. Great for the patient and for the hospital.

Medication education. While hospitals tend to focus on medication reconciliation, the education of patients is often ignored or incomplete. Patients need to understand what they are taking a medication for, the consequences of not taking it, what side effects to look out for, interactions with other medications including over the counter and herbal medicines and what to do if they are going to run out of their medicines. The consequences of not educating patients should be obvious, and a process needs to be in place to ensure they understand their medications before they leave.

Follow-up plans. Many patients need a definitive plan for follow-up with a physician. Appointments need to be made and issues surrounding the patient's ability to get to follow-up appointments must be addressed as well. Home care or other ancillary needs have to be considered. Sub-specialty follow-up can be a significant issue for patients without a PCP and should be arranged in a timely fashion. Most 30-day readmissions (50%) actually occur in the first 2 weeks following discharge and are often related to follow-up issues [21] I was working on an analysis of 30-day readmissions at a hospital I worked for and we discovered that there was a high percentage of cardio-thoracic post-bypass patients that were being readmitted within 30 days. Well over 20%. Diving deeper into the reasons for return, we found that there were 3 outstanding reasons:

(1) A urinary tract infection
(2) Chest pain
(3) Palpitations

We also noted that no patient had been referred to their PCP for follow-up shortly after discharge. We instituted a program to have automated follow-up visits with the primary care doctor within 72 h with a focus on patient education, an office EKG, and an office urinalysis. The program was never instituted due to a hold on all improvement processes because of the implementation of a new electronic health record. I can only hope that at some point after my departure this process improvement plan was put in place and had an impact.

Hand-off. The proper transfer of care to another physician requires a physician-to-physician or provider (NP, PA, MD) hand-off. This is simply the best way to ensure that any given patient's care needs will be met at the time of discharge. This hand-off provides the follow-up provider with information on the patient's diagnosis, treatment rendered, testing completed, sub-specialty consultation obtained and any other outstanding issues such as need for medication adjustment, changes in medications or dosages, and need for further testing and/or consultation.

The patient. Let us not forget that patients have a responsibility for their own healthcare as well. Diabetics who continue to eat whatever they feel like, COPD patients who continue to smoke and patients refusing to take their medications and follow-up, are all more likely to end up back in the ED. Healthcare is a team-based approach and part of that team is the patient. It has always amazed me that citizens are legally required to wear a seatbelt while driving a car, which has been shown to save lives, but motorcycle riders in many states are allowed to ride without a helmet. Those of us in healthcare can do a great deal to improve outcomes for our patients, but we still require the help of our patients to keep themselves healthy and safe.

Patient care does not end when a patient leaves the hospital and neither does the hospital's accountability. CMS is penalizing institutions with high 30-day readmission rates. In addition to this, patient satisfaction surveys are completed after discharge, and will reflect a poor outcome or poor hand-off in many cases. Again, patient satisfaction scores affect reimbursements under Value-Based Care. In these ways, and others, hospitals today are motivated to take better care of patient hand-offs, better educate patients, and better ensure that positive outcomes for their patients are achieved. Standardizing a quality discharge process, therefore, should be far from controversial for any hospital.

The institution of "Bundled Payments" has resulted in hospitals taking on an even larger financial risk with patients. These programs can result in the hospital being responsible for the patient's entire continuum of care for up to 90 days. This includes things such as rehabilitation, homecare, equipment, and readmissions to the hospital. Heath care delivery and risk are driving rapid changes in reimbursement.

Finally, other areas are being monitored for the future. Return visits to the ED within 30 days are being scrutinized. Multiple patient acquired conditions are being monitored such as central line infections or falls. These and others will continue and hopefully the hospitals and staff are receptive to the fact that these things are really in the best interest of patient care, not penalty.

An Emergency Department PCAT Model: The HOT ZONE

The HOT ZONE was a project our team discussed but never had the opportunity to trial. This was an Emergency Department process improvement initiative. The primary idea was to develop a parallel, team-based process for evaluation of ED patients similar to the PCAT process discussed earlier.

Many Emergency Departments provide a type of rapid triage when patients enter the ED via walk-in. This is often referred to as "Provider in Triage" and consists of a Physician or APP providing a rapid assessment of the patient, a cursory exam, and the ordering of tests or initiation of treatment if deemed appropriate. This might include ordering blood work, an x-ray or providing Tylenol for a fever. The purpose of provider in triage was to expedite the evaluation of patients in a timelier manner to reduce overall throughput time. The idea has merit and I can attest to this as I did a two-week trial of provider in triage at one hospital I worked at. I will say that it was grueling 12-h shifts that were virtually non-stop running from 10 am to 10 pm averaging 65 patients seen each shift. The benefit was approximately 18 patients per day were discharged from triage to home. I had 3 rooms, 2 nurses, and a tech during the 12 h.

There is a downside to provider in triage.

(1) Patients evaluated were all walk-ins
(2) There were limitations on what could be ordered test wise
(3) If individuals doing provider in triage did not particularly like it, they would simply send the patient into the ED proper
(4) If not skilled, you could get seriously behind triaging on a busy day

(5) Some ED providers would get upset because either tests were ordered or they felt the tests ordered were insufficient to evaluate the patient's problem

The HOT ZONE concept took a different approach. We wanted the "HOT ZONE" to evaluate all acute patients entering the ED regardless of portal of entry. Ambulance delivery, walk-in, or drop-offs would all be seen in the HOT ZONE. The HOT ZONE was to be an allocated number of beds using a team-based approach for patient evaluations during the busiest periods of ED activity.

Currently, most ED Physicians see on average 1.8 patients per h in the ED. There may be some who see more, or some see less but that is the average. The amount of time an ED provider actually spends with a patient is relatively brief. On average, this is about 8 min. The goal for the HOT ZONE was to design a system that would allow the provider to see over 4 patients per hour. In order to do this, it required the following team members in a 4 bed HOT ZONE—Physician, Nurse, Scribe, Tech, available Respiratory therapist, and Registrar.

The HOT ZONE size will be dependent on the team removing patients quickly after the patient's initial assessment and workup. In the beginning, the maximum time a patient could remain in the HOT ZONE would be 1 h. The patients coming to this zone will have had minimal if any evaluation. Triage would be direct to the zone, rapid registration would be done in the zone, and the ED provider would evaluate and determine testing needs and highest probability disorder in very short order. Lab work would be acquired, EKG, vital signs, and placement of IV and fluids if indicated. Initial treatment would be initiated and if necessary, a patient may require intubation or cardioversion. The only patients not placed here would be patients in acute cardiac arrest; they would be placed in the trauma room because the time allocation could bring the HOT ZONE to a screeching halt.

The key component of this concept was getting all other hospital resources to be active participants. Patients requiring the ICU needed to leave in 1 h, patients requiring an acute procedure like cardiac catheterization needed to leave in 1 h and so on. In addition, once a patient no longer required placement in the HOT ZONE, they would be handed off to another provider. If remaining in the ED, the patient would be handed off to an APP. If the patient clearly required hospital admission, they would be handed off to the receiving hospitalist attending.

The purpose was to take advantage of the unique skill sets of an Emergency Department Physician-Resuscitate-Evaluate-Treat-Disposition. There were many unanswered questions by the team about the concept and how it would function. It clearly required a set volume of patients being evaluated each hour in order to be cost effective and functional. So, this idea might not be usable for very small EDs that see 20 or 30 patients daily and for large EDs may require more than one team to manage the higher volume. Perhaps someone will put the concept to the test in the future.

30-Day Readmission Discussion and Strategies

30-Day readmissions have gotten a lot of press, ever since the passing of the Patient Protection and Affordable Care Act by President Obama on March 23, 2010. In fiscal 2013, Obamacare, as the act has come to be known, initiated significant penalties for hospitals with high 30-day readmission rates—and the department of Health and Human Services announced plans to increase the program to include more patient types in fiscal 2015. Beginning with a 1% reduction in Medicare payments, the penalty quickly ramps up to 3%, and as more patient types are included, the overall risk of losses will grow significantly. In its first year, more than 2,200 hospitals were penalized, with approximately

$280,000,000 in reduced payments. Hospitals are taking notice, and many are implementing strategies to address their readmission issues. We will review some of these approaches and will also look closely at how hospitals can achieve low readmissions—while keeping patient care as their focus, not just government dollars [22]. In 2019, Skilled Nursing Homes have also come under scrutiny for 30-day readmissions. Impacts on reimbursement will be implemented for those nursing homes performing poorly in 2019. Interestingly, for Nursing Homes achieving quality improvement in 30-day readmissions, reward incentives around reimbursement are also being established.

One also must consider how readmissions have traditionally been viewed by hospital administrations across the United States. I once sat in a meeting led by our Chief Financial Officer, whose presentation focused on the positive financial benefits of readmissions. He believed that any government penalties would be offset by readmission revenues—and argued against investing in a readmission reduction program. This viewpoint, which is likely diminishing in the face of a new reality, nevertheless can limit the interest in readmission reduction programs.

30-Day readmissions were expensive and undesirable, however, even before penalties came along. In fact, it is likely that the expense of readmissions led to the penalties in the first place. They cost everyone money, and preventable readmissions represent a failure to care for patients.

From a hospital capacity management standpoint, readmissions are a major problem. Although there are variations caused by numerous factors, on average about 5%–10% of ED patients admitted as an inpatient each day are a 30-day readmission, meaning they were admitted in the prior 30-day period and have returned. A hospital that admits 50 inpatients daily therefore has about 3–5 readmits daily that were just admitted <30 days ago. LOS for readmits is about 6 days.

And preventable readmits (we will go into this further) comprise approximately 20%–40% of all readmissions [23]. Over a year, the volume of preventable readmits at this hospital would be approximately 200–400. With the 6-day LOS, 400 patients would account for 2,400 bed days—a very significant impact on capacity, made even worse by the resulting costs and penalties. Many hospitals in the United States, particularly those serving vulnerable populations, have far higher rates of 30-day readmissions, and will be in serious financial difficulty if they cannot stem the problem—with or without additional penalties.

The term "admitted as an inpatient" contains a very important distinction. Currently, Medicare does not view patients who have been in the hospital as outpatients in this mix. Examples would be patients placed in observation status in the hospital or have been in an extended stay status secondary to some procedure. These patients are exempt from the calculations for 30-day readmission statistics. It is often speculated that this exemption may have resulted in some hospitals classifying large numbers of patients as outpatients as a mechanism to artificially reduce 30-day readmission inpatient rates. I have not read anywhere that this type of gaming is going on. It is likely, however, that CMS will incorporate all types of hospitalizations in their readmission calculations in the future as well as 30-day revisits to the Emergency Department.

In reality, there are readmissions with all types of patient, whether insured or not, beyond even Medicare's vast influence. All of these are expensive. The average "cost" for a hospital surrounding a 30-day readmission is around $10,000 [34]. In this environment, particularly given the additional costs and risks of penalties, hospitals are driving hard to reduce their readmissions. To understand their strategies, it is important to distinguish between the two primary components of the readmission population they wish to reduce.

PPR readmissions. Potentially Preventable Readmissions are patients who are readmitted with the same or similar diagnosis. It is generally understood that if their initial discharge process were handled correctly, this readmission could have been prevented. There is debate about how many readmissions really fit in this category but estimates generally range from 20%–50% of all 30-day readmissions.

Unpreventable readmissions. These are patients discharged from the hospital and readmitted within 30 days with a diagnosis completely unrelated to the primary admission. An example would be a patient admitted with pneumonia who goes home and 3 weeks later gets hit by a car and comes back in as a trauma readmission. These cases make up about 50% of readmissions.

There have been numerous approaches to readmission reduction, in a wide variety of hospitals across the United States. Strategies have varied, according to conditions such as state law, insurance type, and differences in populations.

State Variability

Every state but Maryland will have Medicare reimbursement at acute care hospitals impacted by PPACA. The variability is as follows.

Maryland

The Bay State has a unique reimbursement system. Rates are set for all payers regarding facility fee reimbursement (i.e. -DRG) by a single organization representing hospitals. In 2013, the state's readmissions reimbursement strategy was in operation. Maryland consists of 49 hospitals in two categories—Total Patient Revenue (TPR) and Admission Readmission Reduction (ARR), which, in January 2014, became Geographic Population-based Reimbursement (GPR). TPR hospitals receive a lump sum payment to care for citizens in their defined geographic area. Because TPR hospitals are technically (and realistically) at risk for ALL care delivery, including ALL readmissions, there is no payment on 30-day readmissions to penalize. The ARR model paid hospitals more for initial admissions, in order to offset unpreventable readmission volume. This provided funds for hospitals to actively engage in readmissions reductions programs. This model rewarded hospitals that were able to reduce readmissions. Then in January of 2014, the ARR model was replaced with the GPR model, which is very similar to TPR. These hospitals are also now provided set funds to manage patients within a defined geographic region. The hospitals determine where to focus their spending. This has resulted in a significant interest in reducing readmissions, as well as reducing inpatient and ED utilization. Maryland's model may well replace the current Fee for Service models across the rest of the country and is being watched extremely closely.

Maryland's system also counts any Observation level of care patient that was in the hospital for more than 24 h eligible for the readmission volume if they end up coming back as a 30-day readmission.

49 States

In the rest of the country, 30-day readmissions are handled much differently. PPACA or "Obamacare" has established penalties for acute care hospitals based on readmission rates for a select number of diagnoses. Affected diagnoses have expanded and may do so again. Hospital metrics are weighted and then compared to national performance averages. Poor performance is penalized via a reduction of a percentage of their total Medicare reimbursements. This penalty was quickly ramped up from 1% of all pure Medicare reimbursement in 2013, to 2% in 2014, and 3% in 2015.

Commercial Insurers

Many commercial insurers now deny reimbursement for patients readmitted within 30 days with same or similar conditions. They will review the visits and may opt to combine them in one reimbursement, thus instituting a penalty of sorts. The actual process may vary from state to state, and insurer to insurer, and also vary according to acute care hospital contracts. The reason for this is that many times acute care hospitals and insurers will develop relationships that involve some degree of capitation for a particular population. In effect, this is the same as Maryland's TPR model, but on a smaller scale.

Medicaid

Medicaid reimbursement systems vary widely from state to state. Different states therefore manage 30-day readmission reduction models in very different ways. In some states, there are reviews and denials for payment on patients readmitted within 30 days with same or similar conditions determined by reviewers for the state. The variance in how states handle Medicaid reimbursement for 30-day readmissions is so great that it should suffice to point out that in many places such readmissions are penalized via Medicare, but to varying degrees.

The question underlying all of this is, how can we reduce 30-day readmissions? The fact that hospitals across the country are asking this is itself a movement in the right direction regarding patient care and good management. But which approaches will be effective and sustainable? There are numerous models being evaluated currently, including Project BOOST, Project RED, the STARR Project and the Coleman model to name a few [24–27]. Each has unique attributes and specific goals. Different aspects of hospital care are the focus of reform, such as standardized discharge processes, early follow-up, accurate medication reconciliation, patient education, and improved communication between non-acute care providers (Nursing Homes, Homecare, and Rehab facilities).

Success varies, and has been attributed to the resolution or improvement of a number of key problems, including:

(1) Patient non-compliance
(2) Delayed follow-up appointments
(3) Sub-optimal communication between caregivers (homecare, nursing homes, etc.)
(4) Lack of ED physician engagement
(5) Non-standardized hospital discharge processes
(6) Psychosocial issues related to everything from homelessness and transportation issues to medication acquisition

Many of these models demonstrate improvements, only to see them go back to baseline at the 60-day mark. Some even see increased readmissions at the 1-year mark. Clearly, reducing readmissions is neither simple nor easy. Another challenge is concern over costs when considering changes to infrastructure or process within a hospital system. Also, shifting patients to the outpatient world to avoid readmission penalties may carry its own costs and risks. No one seems to know which approach will be the best.

Yet, despite the variety of programs already running, they all have one or more primary components in common. Chief among these are standardization and communication. Below is a discussion of each of these, as well as other core components. Successful models will likely vary, according to the individual situations and needs of each hospital. But understanding these core components will be essential for success.

We have seen (and implemented) successful readmission reduction programs, particularly in the state of Maryland. The model below assumes that any patient can be at risk for a 30-day readmission, some more than others based on disease process, support systems and adequate access to healthcare in their community. We'll look at five primary components of a readmission's reduction program, beginning with the PCP.

Role of the PCP in 30-Day Readmission Reduction

PCPs, otherwise known as general practitioners, or in times past referred to as the family doctor, are central to the health care delivery for most patients. These doctors provide regular checkups and preventative health care as well as referrals to specialists and the utilization of acute health care facilities when needed.

It is sometimes pointed out that the best way to reduce readmissions is to prevent admissions in the first place. Routine physicals, HbA1C levels, Blood pressure monitoring, EKGs, cholesterol monitoring, education, and lifestyle counseling are all essential elements of the PCP's mission to prevent sickness. These routine, standard efforts should help prevent onset of disease or determine need for early intervention. The frequency and nature of PCP visits will vary according to each patient's needs and condition. A healthy patient with minimal risks may need no more than an annual physical, while the COPD or CHF patient may require a visit every month. Patients with complex chronic diseases must be adequately monitored. Failure to do so increases the burden placed on acute care facilities and further involves specialty services.

Many specialists are available for referral from the PCP. Often, they are an adjunct to the preventative health care mission. A gastroenterologist performs routine colonoscopies, for example, or a cardiologist might test and evaluate a patient reporting chest pain. Specialists also play a role in the world of acute care, either with elective procedures, such as hip or knee replacement, or with emergency intervention when a patient is stricken with appendicitis or cholecystitis. Most often, these interventions involve a trip to the Emergency Department. Patients with good monitoring, preventative care, healthy lifestyles, and early interventions are less likely to be the cause of a readmission.

I remember doing an analysis of each PCP's 30-day readmission rate at a hospital I worked at. What amazed me was the marked interest physicians had in their particular rate. Physicians are a highly competitive group of individuals. Providing them valid, accurate data on their performance is extremely important in getting changes in behavior. An example is a follow-up visit for a PCP's patient who was in the hospital for 4 or 5 days. Trying to fit this patient into a packed schedule for a 15-min visit will do little to impact a readmission. Patients may have had multiple medication changes or other identified issues that require more investigative follow-up than a 15 min how are you doing kind of visit.

Role of the Emergency Department in 30-Day Readmission Reduction

If you asked most ED providers what their role in 30-day readmissions was, you would probably get a blank stare. While the majority of readmissions come through the ED, the providers there are focused on caring for their patients in a limited time, and with a limited amount of background information. Most of the time, they are unaware that a patient either is a readmission or is at risk of becoming one.

While most readmissions have a PCP, that physician is usually not involved when they enter the ED. Some patients enter the ED while in the care of a specialist. Patients undergoing operations or a Cath, or who were admitted to the care of a psychiatrist may end up in the ED without the knowledge of their PCP. Other patients may come from nursing homes, rehab centers, group homes, homeless shelters, home care agencies, or even prison. Whether or not these patients have a PCP, they arrive in the ED without medical records or a handoff from a PCP. Instead, the ED providers have, on average, about 180 min or less to evaluate, treat, and decide how to disposition each patient. There's little time to search for background information, much less to connect with PCPs. This disconnect between primary care and emergency care is a major cause of the readmission problem.

The disposition options available to most ED physicians are:

(a) Treat and release
(b) Hospitalize
    a. ICU
    b. Acute med/surg
    c. Observation
(c) Transfer to alternate facility

It is fairly rare for a PCP to be available or consulted in this process, a fact which results in higher readmission rates due to lack of background information and knowledge on the part of ED providers.

A few simple changes to the ED process—and provider expectations, can have an impact on these types of readmission risks. Currently, ED providers have no idea whether the patient they are seeing was an inpatient admission in the last 30 days. Because of this, they disposition the patient regardless of this crucial fact, possibly impacting quality of care and outcome, and at the very least a loss of revenue. Obviously, this information is of little consequence when dispositioning an acute life-threatening event. But even in extreme cases, the awareness of prior admits can be important to quality of care and disposition decision making. For example, a physician would want to know that a myocardial infarction patient was recently admitted for a cardiac event.

With today's electronic records, it is possible for ED practitioners to be supplied with admission histories and even medical background information of incoming patients. With this information, providers can consider a range of options to better disposition 30-day readmission patients and may better be able to care for patients at risk of becoming a readmission.

Once the ED provider is aware that the patient they are seeing is indeed someone who had an inpatient admission within the last 30 days, the provider can consider the best disposition for that patient while minimizing the impact of the readmission.

They can consider additional options:

- Treat and Release—provider contacts the PCP to ensure a timely follow-up or, if there is no PCP, arranges to provide one
- Acute Emergent Inpatient—provider contacts the PCP to update patient's status and expected length of stay.
- Non-emergent Hospitalization:
  1. Nursing Home Placement—If the patient is on Medicare and had an inpatient hospital admission in the last 30 days, the patient already satisfies the eligibility criteria for NH placement. Commercial payers will often authorize these transfers. A Social worker or care management assistance may be needed to arrange acceptance, transfer, etc. Examples of patients that may be eligible would be patients with COPD, CHF, or uncontrolled diabetes. PCP contact is again an important component here.
  2. Observation—Patients that need hospitalization but are ineligible for transfer to a NH and do not meet defined criteria (InterQual or Milliman) for acute inpatient admission after review, are best managed in a closed observation unit with appropriate staffing and resources. Even patients with a prior related admission in the last 30 days will be authorized for this type of hospital stay. The PCP is updated on the patient's status and expected length of stay.

3. Patients eligible for inpatient med/surg hospitalization based on InterQual or Milliman criteria. PCP contact to inform them of the plan and status.

The Admitting Process Role in 30-Day Readmissions

As part of an effort to reduce 30-day readmissions, two questions must be addressed when a patient enters the ED. The first is whether the patient had an inpatient admission within the last 30 days and the second is whether the patient is a risk of becoming a readmission in the next 30 days after discharge. This information should be available to the admitting ED provider.

As outlined above, the type of hospitalization that is appropriate for readmission patients must also be considered. Observation patients are not considered readmissions. However, even these patients may be at risk of becoming a readmission upon discharge. The use of a PCAT model is one method to attempt early recognition of a 30-day readmission or a patient at risk for readmission, with provider, nursing, pharmacists, and support all involved at this early stage. The team-based care delivery model provides focus all the way through to the patient discharge to make sure proper follow-up and an ability to address other issues such as medications or transportation.

Standard practice for patient admissions to a hospital unit can easily be checklist-based system:

(1) Anticipated discharge location—home-NH-Rehab, etc.
(2) Transportation needs---family, friends, taxi, stretcher, etc.
(3) Medication needs—insurance, available financial resources, etc.
(4) Anticipated home needs---equipment, oxygen, PT, home care
(5) Follow-up needs----PCP availability, sub-specialty needs, etc.

Asking these questions at the time of admission, will help providers address potential readmission issues prior to their discharge. These components are the starting point. At the time of discharge, additional information will be required. Several variations of this concept are in use today [24].

Patients who have returned to the hospital within 30 days obviously need to be identified and properly dispositioned. But the identification of patients at risk for readmission is more complex. Certain disease processes have been identified as potentially high readmission risk areas:

- CHF
- COPD
- Pneumonia
- Post-sepsis
- Post-acute MI
- Cancer undergoing treatment

Patients who present to the Emergency Department with these diagnoses should be managed in the same fashion as a known 30-day readmission. Once a patient has been identified as either a 30-day readmission or a high risk for readmission and requires inpatient hospitalization, they are transferred to an inpatient bed on a hospital floor, where further processes and considerations must be in place.

The Care Delivery Process

If the hospital unit has no idea the patient is a 30-day readmission or at high risk for readmission, then nothing will change regarding care delivery. Communication from the ED is essential and can be achieved in numerous ways:

- Identification on the unit census board
- Identification on an electronic census board
- Identification within the medical record if paper-based

This forward communication gets the treatment team on the same page. Each member will have a role impacting the patient's likelihood of being readmitted.

The Patient. It is important to ensure that patients understand what may have resulted in their own readmission. A discussion of their recent hospitalization history and health care needs can reduce their risks.

Nurses. Nurses are responsible for educating the patient on their disease process and discussing their role in their own care.

Pharmacy. The patient should receive medication education, including information on accessing and utilizing their medications.

Care Manager/Social Work. These professionals can identify any barriers to care and begin processes to deal with them. These barriers may include transportation, housing, ability to purchase medications, follow-up appointments, etc.

Physician. In addition to educating the patient on disease management, the physician should provide referrals to appropriate outpatient providers—PCP, Sub-specialists, diagnostic testing, lab studies, etc.

Ancillary. These may be representatives of specialty services that can assist in the patient's condition—pulmonary rehab for COPD, CHF clinics, Palliative Care, IT for patients getting computer assist devices to manage their condition, nursing home representatives for patients requiring rehab or longer term placement, diabetic teaching, physical therapy, Home Care, and others, all of whom will impact the patient's care when they leave the acute care facility.

Each facility's resources and capabilities will determine how these team members will interface with patients, but it is essential they do so on day one of every admission. Addressing these issues early reduces LOS and readmission rates, improves discharges before noon, and enhances patient satisfaction. Most acute care patients cycle out of the facility in three days, receiving ongoing care in lower acuity environments, such as transitional care, nursing home, rehab, home with homecare, etc.

A common problem faced by many hospitals is that this process becomes interrupted on weekends and holidays—about 30% of the days of the year. Many ancillary staff are not available, certain testing is unavailable, ability to make follow-up appointments may be limited, and access to transportation options may be limited, and many nursing homes and home care providers are resistant to taking patients over the weekend. Subspecialty consultation and follow-up may be limited, as well, while care managers, social workers, pharmacists, ancillaries, and even physicians are stretched by staffing shortages during these times. Administrations that are committed to reducing 30-day readmissions will require considerable creativity to address this reality—but in a healthcare system that places the highest priority on patient care, it must be addressed.

The Discharge Process Role in 30-Day Readmission Reduction

Simple communication is central to successful reductions of readmissions. By the time of discharge, the patient must be aware of what is happening. They should know when they are leaving, and have any issues related to their transportation and ongoing care addressed in advance. Simply meeting these needs has been shown to improve outcomes, and of course, reduce 30-day readmission rates [35].

Key considerations for any successful program will be:

Disease education. This is usually a cross-functional effort, aimed at ensuring every patient fully understands their healthcare requirements and understands their own role in their recovery or management. A newly diagnosed diabetic without insurance or a PCP will need education, medication, dietary instruction, and a follow-up Physician, for example. This patient will need input from nursing, physician, social work, pharmacy, and a diabetic teacher. Whether the patient smokes or drinks will also be a factor, potentially adding further to the educational component.

Medication education. Incredibly, this is often neglected. Often, patients are sent home with little understanding of the medication they have been prescribed—and can end up right back in the ED as a result. While medication reconciliation may occur, hospitals often fail to go further. Patients need to understand what they are taking a medication for, the consequences of not taking it, what side effects to look out for, interactions with other medications including over the counter and herbal medicines and what to do if you are going to run out of your medicines.

Follow-Up Plans

Before discharge, the hospital should ensure each patient has a solid plan for follow-up with a physician. Appointments need to be made and any transportation issues resolved. Home care or other ancillary needs have to be addressed. Sub-specialty follow-up can be a significant issue for patients without a PCP and should be addressed before discharge. Most 30-day readmissions (50%) actually occur in the first 2 weeks following discharge and are often related to lack of follow-up. High-risk patients should be provided follow-up appointments within 48–72 h following discharge from the acute care facility. As discussed earlier, when we surveyed PCPs about follow-up appointments for their patients following a hospitalization, the majority of time the patient was added onto the doctor's already busy schedule resulting in a 10- or 15-min visit. Patients with complex diseases, multiple medications, and extended stays in the hospital will usually require a much longer appointment visit to make sure all the patients' issues are addressed.

Hand-off. Physician to physician hand-offs, or Provider to Provider if PAs or NPs are utilized ensure that further care needs will be met at the time of discharge. This provides the follow-up provider with information on the patient's diagnosis, treatment rendered, testing completed, sub-specialty consultation obtained and any other outstanding issues such as need for medication adjustment, changes in medications or dosages, and need for further testing and/or consultation.

Addressing these issues at discharge will result in all members of the patient's healthcare team, both hospital-based and non-hospital-based, to be on the same page in understanding what the needs of the patient will be, and ensure the patients themselves understand their own condition and care needs. Communication at this level has become vital as our healthcare delivery system has grown ever more fragmented. Hospitals that educate patients and coordinate with PCPs will certainly see fewer of their patients return within 30 days. If, however, the PCP is unaware of the patient's current hospitalization, care rendered, medication changes, referral to an alternative care facility, sub-specialty consultation, testing or use of home care, then a very high rate of 30-day readmissions is inevitable.

Certain specialty surgical procedures have been shown to have a high rate of 30-day readmissions. In particular, post-CABG, post-Vascular, and post-Colorectal surgeries experience readmission problems. Why is this? Because of lack of follow-up and communication with PCPs. Often, secondary issues that could have been foreseen or adverted with proper communication and follow-up cause readmissions—and patients are rarely admitted to the surgical service they were discharged from. Instead they flow back to the ED. Many of these patients have medical issues that the PCP is skilled at managing. These medical issues can become complicated in surgical patients that have diabetes, heart disease or multiple other medical disorders.

A typical example of this phenomenon, which was discussed earlier, would be a post-CABG patient experiencing chest pain or palpitations, developing a fever or UTI or have some other condition which may be linked to the surgery itself. Timely follow-up with that patient's PCP before initial discharge would likely result in a standard post-CABG protocol, including items such as EKG, U/A, physical exam, and education, all of which would reduce the chances significantly of a readmission—while improving the chances of a positive outcome for the patient.

Models for facilitating this level of communication and follow-up will vary, but should include hard hand offs, follow-up appointments and education. Any hospital interested in reducing readmissions (and caring for patients) must address this need.

The Post Discharge Role in 30-Day Readmission Reductions

Patients are discharged to a variety of settings when leaving acute care:

(1) Nursing home
(2) Skilled rehab
(3) Alternate facility-(Psych), group home, prison
(4) Shelter
(5) Home
(6) Hospice

Discharged patients are also referred to a variety of providers. Some common referrals are:

(1) Home care
(2) Physical therapy
(3) Respiratory therapy

(4) Diabetic teaching
(5) Home visit provider-physician or APP

Regardless of what facility or provider is involved, the PCP needs to be aware of where their patient is and who is caring for them. The importance of this cannot be understated. Many patients return to the ED because of a lack of communication with the PCP at discharge and when a referral occurs. Often, a home care visit results in a readmission, with no communication with or direction from a poorly informed and unaware PCP. Without the opportunity to properly care for this patient, the PCP is rendered useless and the patient's chance for a positive outcome is diminished.

There is no doubt that 30-day readmission reductions can have a significant impact on hospital capacity management, as well as on hospital finances. We recommend that hospitals develop broadly represented 30-day readmission reduction committees. While a challenge to administer, this area of healthcare will only become more important in years to come, as the transition of care to the outpatient arena becomes more prominent and as CMS continues to increase penalties for high readmissions rates. Healthcare organizations that develop quality discharge policies now will reap rewards well into the future and will provide better quality and lower cost care for their patients.

Chapter 12

Additional Capacity Management Programs

Proceduralist Program

Another program that a hospital can consider is a Proceduralist program. The concept of this program is to provide a trained team of APPs (NPs and PAs) to provide a flexible and efficient method to have various vascular lines placed or certain procedures done. The current method of acquiring the placement of vascular lines and procedures is to use a combination of resources whose availability may be spotty at best. Having an identified trained individual available for this purpose could have a significant impact on patient length of stay, efficiency of procedure acquisition or vascular line placement, improved patient safety and improved patient, and staff satisfaction.

I can remember when I was in training for my Internal Medicine residency, we were required to perform all the procedures and line placements in the hospital. This included the following:

(1) Central line placement
(2) Difficult peripheral line placement

(3) Arterial line placement
(4) Thoracentesis
(5) Paracentesis
(6) Lumbar puncture

There was limited ability of radiology, phlebotomy, or surgery to provide these services. Things have changed dramatically over the last 34 years. Rarely do residents perform procedures or place lines and the result is to schedule a patient through interventional radiology or perhaps get an intensivist, neurologist, or surgeon to assist in some of the procedures. The result can be significant delays in the line being placed or the procedure being performed. This adds to the patients' LOS on many occasions or at a minimum, less satisfied patients who may have to wait for extended periods to get the procedure done. The implementation of a proceduralist program could mitigate those issues. The program would pay for the APP by billing professional fees for the procedures performed.

The following benefits to the program could be experienced:

Efficiency—Patients would have procedures done in a more efficient manner by having specific staff trained in invasive procedures. The more procedures a provider undertakes, the more skilled and efficient the provider becomes.

Utilization management—Patients many times may have the wrong type of line placed. By having trained proceduralists, patients would get the right line the first time. Inappropriate use of PICC lines would decrease. Trying to manage patients with inadequate peripheral lines would be resolved.

Revenue generation—Currently, many of the invasive procedures are not billed by providers. Each procedure has a separate CPT code and an associated professional fee and facility fee attached to it. By properly billing for procedures, many hospitals have found that the cost for the proceduralist group can be adequately covered by professional fee billing.

Patient safety—By having a trained team of proceduralists, the complication rate for invasive procedures has been found to be less than 1% compared with 2%–5% nationally. Strict adherence to infection control techniques would be standardized with a proceduralist team.

Reduced length of stay—Since the proceduralist group would be available 24/7, patients would no longer be awaiting a procedure, for example, in interventional radiology. Such patients may have a shorted length of stay by getting procedures done in a timely fashion.

Medical staff satisfaction—Clearly, medical staff members whose skill sets are no longer adequately maintained for invasive procedures would have a defined team to provide the services necessary for the care of their patients in a timely fashion which will significantly improve physician satisfaction.

Additional types of services could be rendered to provide sufficient procedure volume for the APP. This could include:

(1) PICC lines
(2) Dialysis catheters
(3) Tunnel catheters
(4) G-tube replacement
(5) Suprapubic catheters

There are likely additional procedures that could be performed. The APP would be under the supervision of an attending physician in the main hospital. Impact on overall LOS would vary depending on the overall volume of procedures done, the current procedure wait time, and the impact a proceduralist would have. The impact would be most evident on the weekends when many times, a patient will wait the entire weekend for a procedure on Monday because the procedure was not deemed to be emergent.

Chapter 13

Discharges before Noon

A key aspect of hospital capacity management, which is often studied and written about, is the problem of late discharges causing capacity bottlenecks. Getting patients discharged, and making their beds available, before noon each day (therefore beating the rush of afternoon and evening admissions) is a goal for many hospitals. In a hospital running extremely high census numbers and basically starting the day with a significant bed deficit, there is a need to acquire some breathing room to accommodate the influx of additional admissions through the ED and directs and transfers. This is really the driving force behind discharges before noon.

As we touched on in the previous chapter, there is plenty of variance in how hospitals process discharges in the first place. And there are many different definitions of what constitutes a discharge, as previously discussed. The already complex process of discharge is often delayed when different departments and team members fail to communicate and lack a standardized process. Discharge information, if not quickly and easily accessible to bed-assignment, results in cleaned beds sitting empty for significant periods of time. This simple problem is so prevalent in some organizations that individuals are assigned to walk through the hospital to determine if there are any available cleaned beds. In some cases, departments have been known to hide beds and deliberately delay inputs into the electronic system, causing trust issues between different hospital units, not to mention capacity management headaches. Many times, secretarial input is required to remove the patient from the electronic system but is delayed because the secretary has prioritized other duties or is on break or at lunch thus delaying the necessary up to date information to bed assignment. This alone can cause major capacity management problems.

The definition I like best for patient discharge is the time the bed is available for the next patient. This time should be placed into the system in some manner by environmental services when the bed clean is completed. The other definitions are really pending discharges.

On a number of hospital consultations, I have encountered incentive programs designed to speed patient discharges. However, upon close inspection, I have found that sometimes these programs can actually worsen the problem. In one case, when incentivized on a daily basis, hospitalists would keep patients until the next day in order to game the system and achieve a higher discharge before noon rate. Incentives clearly need to be broader than any one component of capacity management. Linking early discharges with improved LOS and 30-day readmission metrics, for example, will help to drive real improvements and encourage everyone to think in terms of what's best for patients and the hospital. Hospitals have resorted to all sorts of signage to clarify to patients the expected discharge time. "Discharge is to Occur by 11 am" or some other notice placed in the patient's room. The concept of having the hospital function similar to a hotel is nice but not at all realistic. The purpose of discharges before noon in a hotel is to allow prep time of the room for the next guest check-in at 3 pm. The purpose in the hospital is also to provide patient entry into the room. The biggest difference is the hospital has patients waiting for rooms well before "3 pm check-in." There may be admitted boarders sitting in the Emergency Department, the operating rooms started at 7 am and have patients in the PACU awaiting beds and the Cath lab has been running and may well need beds available to them. This demand/capacity mismatch (demonstrated in Figures 13.1 and 13.2) is a primary barrier to the movement of patients and another key component to capacity management.

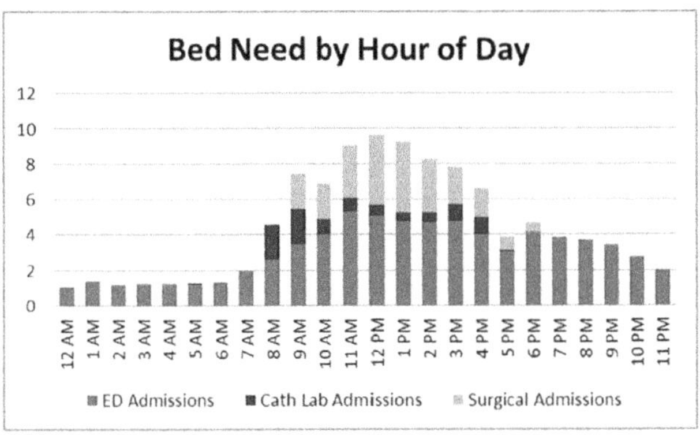

Figure 13.1 A Western NY 500-bed hospital's average daily bed need all demand streams.

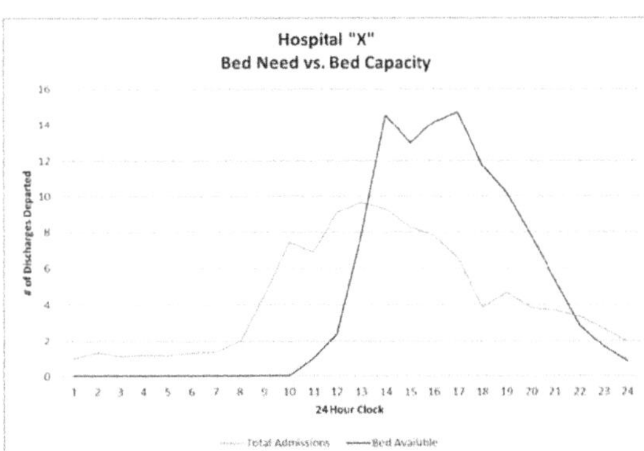

Figure 13.2 Mismatch of bed available by hour with actual hour patient needs bed.

This mismatch can have serious consequences for patient movement out of various areas of the hospital resulting in excessive boarding hours in the Emergency Department, impact environmental service staffing levels, and impact workload on nursing staff on the various units.

Admissions are much more time consuming than discharges from a nursing perspective and can create significant workload issues. One method to manage that workload problem was the previously discussed PCAT's team in which head to toe nursing assessments would be done at the time of admission in the ED. There are other workload issues which will affect discharge effectiveness:

Physicians

They need to know when discharges are a high priority, and also need to communicate with the patient and family when discharge is pending. They also need to communicate to nurses. Simply entering a discharge order is not an effective method of communication. It was routine when I would ask about the discharge process in various hospitals that I would be told by physicians that they did an awesome job of writing discharge orders before noon. Then I would have a discussion with the nursing staff who said they had no idea when a discharge order had been written and received no verbal communication from the provider. I referred to it as a secret discharge.

Secretaries

They must remove patients from the census in a timely fashion and immediately communicate with bed-assignment and environmental services. This may involve coverage for breaks and lunch, etc.

Nurses

They need to know if decisions are being made which will affect environmental services staffing, such as intra-unit transfers or patients going for testing for example.

Bed-Assignment

They need to know if there is sufficient staffing to manage the demand of multiple admissions coming from various areas with different needs during peak demand times.

Environmental Services

Must assign sufficient staffing to meet the demand of bed cleans. Newer cleaning methodologies have resulted in longer clean times for rooms resulting in extended bed turn-over times. This means that a standard of 30 min per bed clean may now come close to 1 h or longer for what are referred to as "terminal cleans" (Figure 13.3).

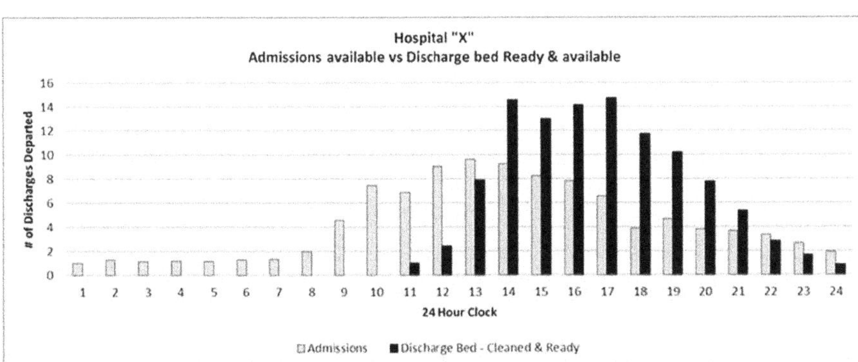

Figure 13.3 Example of timing of admissions versus bed available time.

Any given hospital will need to understand how many discharges before noon are required and will need to develop a plan to achieve that objective.

The question of how many discharges before noon is based on a number of factors.

Hospital Occupancy

A hospital with relatively low occupancy and multiple beds available to patients has little need for discharges before noon from a patient flow perspective. However, from a staffing and cost perspective, managing discharges well could have a major impact. How many hospitals can afford to maintain a significant number of empty beds to deal with the natural and artificial variability created by the ED, OR, and Cath labs? Staffing up and down for various scenarios can be challenging to say the least. The primary use of hospital capacity management is to manage the demand/capacity needs of the hospital at the lowest cost and the highest efficiency and most significant value to the patient. This requires even small, lower occupancy hospitals to be good at capacity management.

Leveling

The concept of leveling has been written about extensively. Leveling is the process of managing artificial variability. Artificial variability is the ebb and flow of admissions created by a process that is controlled and managed. The elective OR and Cath lab schedules are good examples of this. The idea is to distribute this scheduled volume equally throughout the week so that peaks and troughs do not occur and the ability to predict and manage this portion of overall demand becomes much easier.

Leveling has proven difficult to implement. Many facilities have attempted what I refer to as part-time leveling, trying to level cases Monday through Friday. The purest form of leveling would be managing cases 7 days a week. But, as discussed in earlier sections, even these part-time attempts rarely succeed. Discharges before noon is simply an easier way to manage variability. Why? Well, it does not cost as much in political capital to institute. This is not to imply that leveling as a component of capacity management should not be attempted, it is just that the ability to effectively implement leveling requires an extremely mature organization and a profound change in physician behavior.

Provider Staffing

In hospitals without hospitalist services, the decision to discharge is usually made at the time rounds are conducted. This is predominantly in the morning hours. Therefore, any pending studies that day will be missed, and those patients will stay an extra night. Weekend rounding by private internists usually occurs later in the morning. Because these are usually covering physicians, and not the patient's primary physician, they are less likely to make discharge decisions. Vacations and holidays pose an additional problem.

In the Hospitalist world it is slightly different. The primary issues here are related to priority rounding, geographic staffing, and level staffing. Clearly, the sickest patient assigned to the hospitalist should be seen first. The second priority should be patients eligible for discharge that day. If done properly the patient has already been prepared and prepped for discharge so the process should be seamless. The issues with geographic staffing come into play when the hospitalist has patients on multiple units throughout the hospital. The impact of this was discussed in the "Team-Based Care" section in Chapter 11.

Non-leveled staffing also causes issues, as reduced weekend staffing results in reduced discharges. Finally, hospitalist changeovers cause delays in discharges. Most of the time the new team is trying to learn the patients and their problems—and not prioritizing discharges. This is a side effect of the electronic hand-offs in the new world of medicine.

Testing and Consulting

These are two areas that obviously can have impact based on when the test has been done and read or when a consultant has provided input on a patient. Even if testing is done in a timely fashion, the reading of the test may well be the rate-limiting step. This is classic with radiology and cardiology. Patients receive a study and there is no priority placed on reading the study and it gets into a queue with the rest of the studies. The result is a delay in the read, and a delay in discharge.

If we now look at the overall discharge volume by day of week as shown below, we can determine that on average we need 38 discharges in our Hospital before noon, to satisfy the input variables. This includes ED admits, OR admits, and Cath lab admits. So for our example, we would estimate that our facility needs 35% of discharges before noon to satisfy the demand. The sweet spot for discharges before noon is usually around the 30% mark which satisfies most organizations demand needs in the early part of the day. This then allows the ED, OR, and Cath lab to decompress and manage the remaining cases and admissions continuing to come through those portals (Figure 13.4).

Approximately 17 beds would be freed up before noon just by increasing the number of discharges by noon to 30%. For many hospitals, this is all it would take to resolve capacity management woes throughout each day.

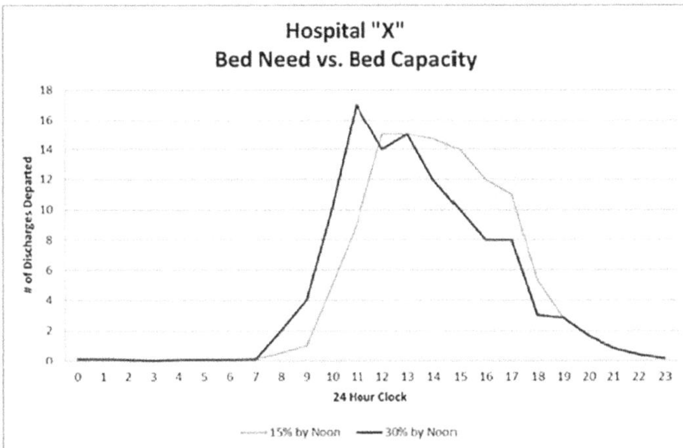

Figure 13.4 The capacity gained by shifting the departure curve from 15% by noon to 30%.

Achieving Discharges before Noon

To succeed, everyone involved in the discharge process must be held to a single standardized process and comply with it. Those standards should be present on every hospital unit, especially the medical units since medical discharges are the cause of most delays. The first step is clarifying the definition of a discharge.

Discharge Definition: The Patient Has Left the Bed, The Bed Has Been Cleaned, and Notification Has Reached Bed Assignment

With this definition established, a process to improve discharges before noon can be developed. Variations, of course, will be dictated by factors unique to each facility, such as provider staffing variability and hospital occupancy, but the underlying elements, such as the establishment of great communication, should be the same everywhere.

Communication between hospital personnel takes one of two forms: face-to-face and electronic. Each has its strengths and weaknesses. Face-to-face is certainly preferable when providers communicate an order for a patient, for example. But discharge requires the involvement of multiple individuals. For effective discharge before noon programs, electronic communications will be essential. Many forms of electronic communications are available, from email and text to cell-phone calls and intranet services. But in our experience, the electronic census board is best, for the following reasons:

(1) It is a central point of communication for multiple metrics—Length of Stay, Use of Telemetry, Census on Floor, Discharge, Readmission, and many others
(2) Everyone can see the status of the unit and determine their next priority, be it environmental services, consultants, providers, etc.
(3) Visual cues, such as color codes, can be employed. This is a very simple, highly effective means to communicate escalations, such as when certain time spans have elapsed from discharge order to bed cleaning: Green for 30 min, yellow for 1 h and red for greater than 1 h.
(4) The board is always updated so whenever information is viewed it is real time
(5) Linkage to bed assignment allows better management of bed capacity in the organization
(6) Parameters can be defined, such as acceptable number of patients on telemetry. The board can warn of impending crises and help trigger appropriate measures, such as, in this case, reviewing telemetry patients to determine who can be removed from telemetry
(7) Readmitted patients can be flagged as high risk during the discharge process
(8) Eliminates the need for bed czars walking through the hospital trying to find an empty bed
(9) Can Flag patients with pending tests

There are likely other electronic systems, but this approach has been proven effective. The point is to implement a robust, centralized system of communicating in real time to everyone in the hospital who needs to stay informed. Census boards certainly work extremely well in the ED, giving up to the minute information to everyone on vital signs, status of labs, radiographs, medication delivery, and EKG's. All important information to track and maintain that 3-h treatment and disposition window. The days of whiteboards and erasers are behind us.

The standard work that refines the discharge process follows. This standard work should be a daily routine by each individual involved in the discharge process (Table 13.1).

Table 13.1 Discharge Process

STANDARD WORK: DISCHARGE CHECKLIST TO BE COMPLETED BY DISCHARGE NURSE OR SOCIAL WORKER			
DATE:	*Pt Name:*	*Contact Name*	*Ph#*
Y/N		*COMMENTS*	
	Home Oxygen?		
	Ride home on discharge day?		
	Clothing to wear home?		
	Keys to your residence?		
	Able to obtain prescriptions?		
	Approval received for all new medications?		
	Equipment ready at home?		
	Patient's family understands diagnosis and treatment?		
	All high risk medications have been reviewed		
	Medication reconciliation with pre-admission list		
	SNF Provider has been contacted?		

Standardization during Discharge

A standardized discharge process that will work as follows with transport and environmental services: All patients discharged home will be picked up by transport which will be activated by unit-based nursing. Transport will stop at the secretarial desk of the unit and inform the secretary to remove the patient from the unit census. Transport will also activate environmental services that the room requires cleaning. Information provided would expect to reduce LOS of discharged patients by 5 h per patient. This would likely improve discharge volumes earlier in the day (goal would be 30%) impacting LOS of ED admitted patients. EMS picking up discharges should be to sign into the nursing station before and after acquiring the patient for discharge. The unit secretary should remove the patient from the system and activate environmental services. A unit log could be used to track time frames and hold secretarial staff accountable for this task.

Chapter 14

Leveling

Throughout this book are references to leveling. No discussion of hospital capacity management can really be considered complete without addressing this concept—and looking closely at how it might be executed in practice. Leveling, if achieved, allows for increased capacity in two different ways:

(1) It creates capacity for growing specialty lines by providing optimal utilization of specialty rooms or equipment
(2) It creates hospital capacity by reducing the overall volume of inpatient beds needed to service a particular surgical specialty or service line

As discussed in other chapters, leveling is the management of artificial variability in any given process. Natural variability is what we usually think of as variability inherent to healthcare with the most frequent example cited being the Emergency Department. Artificial variability is the variability we impose on ourselves through scheduled procedures, day to day, and hour to hour. The best example is the Operating Room. Patients are scheduled for surgery weeks, if not months in advance of their procedure. Artificial variability is created by the resulting schedule of various procedures. Because the scheduling is based on provider allocated Operating Room time, special room or equipment availability, and the providers work schedule outside the Operating Room, the resulting schedules often vary greatly in volume from day to day.

Leveling limits this variability by equally spreading out the different surgical procedures over a period of time. Ideally, this would be 7 days a week, but most hospitals still operate on a Monday through Friday schedule, which still produces a significant amount of artificial variability.

In order to closely examine and understand how Leveling works (and does not, as the case may be) we will take a look at a typical example of Leveling below. You will see that this is an extremely difficult process to master and implement in a busy Operating Room with multiple specialties. But you should also see that Leveling can make a very significant difference in hospital capacity management, and can be achieved, if approached correctly and with the right amount of dedication to making it happen.

Leveling an Orthopedics Service Line

Orthopedic surgery provides an excellent example when demonstrating the leveling process. When looking at the overall surgical schedule a number of components must be taken into account. Operating Rooms are not solely for patients requiring an extended inpatient admission. The Operating Room schedule will have a number of different kinds of patients scheduled for procedures:

(1) Patients with procedures requiring an inpatient hospitalization.
(2) Patients with procedures that may require an extended stay in the hospital but not be considered

inpatients—patients with refractory vomiting after a procedure, for example

(3) Patients with procedures that will be discharged to home after the procedure

These patient types are important because they present a variety of acuity. Scheduling a high percentage of low acuity cases on one day and a large number of high acuity patients requiring hospitalization on another can have a significant impact on overall capacity management. Leveling is more complex than just scheduling the same volume of cases daily throughout the week. It is also necessary to understand the length of stay of those patients requiring hospitalization. Various procedures will require different lengths of stay in an organization depending on the complexity of the procedure, complications following the procedure, the patients' co-morbidities and ability to improve after the procedure, and availability of ancillary staff and resources to manage the patient after the procedure. A standard hip replacement length of stay is approximately 3 days, for example. Most of these patients require some type of onsite rehab and offsite rehab following the procedure. If the patient's procedure is scheduled on Friday, then physical therapy must be available in the hospital over the weekend to provide the rehab initiation. If scheduled on Thursday, the patient may require home physical therapy or transfer to a rehab facility that must be willing to accept the patient on the weekend. These become overly complex systems issues which can have an extraordinary impact on the entire hospital system's ability to manage capacity and level the Operating Room (Figures 14.1 and 14.2).

Looking at the orthopedic surgery example in more detail reveals what the successful leveling of one single specialty could impact. Looking at graphs from an actual hospital in New York, we can first see the three types of patients

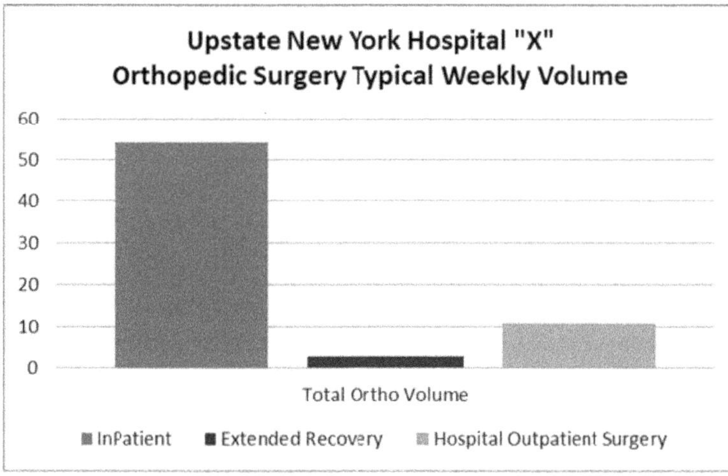

Figure 14.1 Typical orthopedic surgical week in Upstate New York.

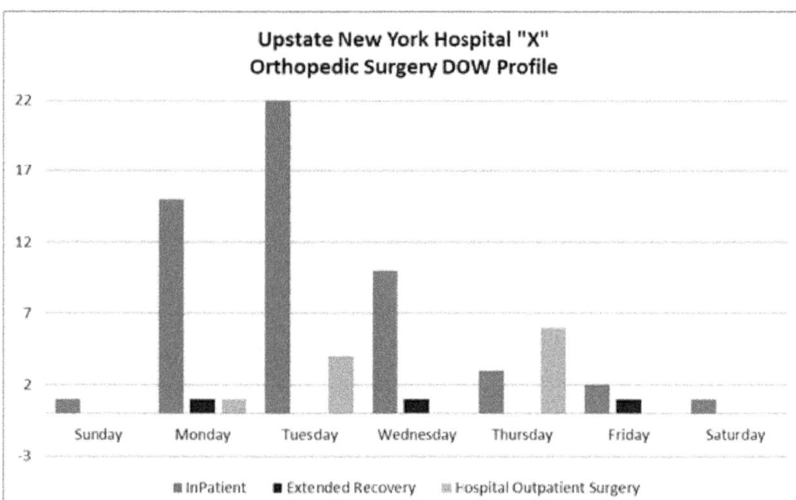

Figure 14.2 Orthopedic surgical DOW profile.

scheduled throughout the week for a high orthopedic volume facility. Clearly, inpatient procedures are dominant.

The graph above demonstrates a breakdown of these same orthopedic cases by day of the week. Notice the high volume of inpatient cases scheduled for Monday and Tuesday and how volume tapers off by the end of the week.

This demonstrates the daily bed need for the population being scheduled. The next graph simply extrapolates the number of new beds this orthopedic volume will require each day (Figure 14.3).

What we see here does not yet accurately represent bed need because we have yet to factor in length of stay. If we agree that the extended stay cases will only require 1 bed day and the inpatient procedure patients will require 3 bed days, our graph for bed need changes dramatically, as seen in the graph below in Figure 14.4.

With this degree of bed need variability, the need for leveling becomes clear. By leveling bed need and factoring in

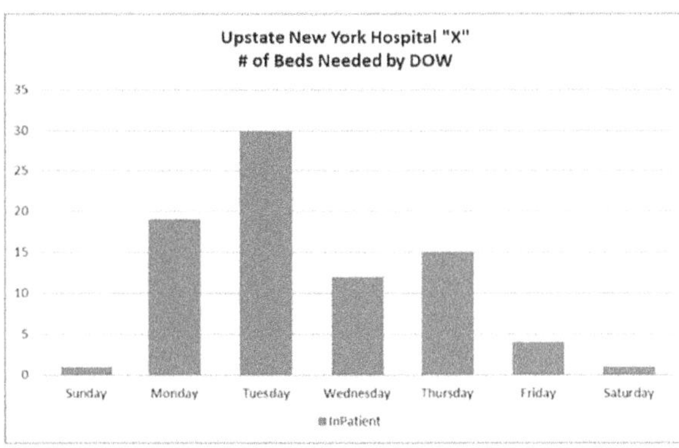

Figure 14.3 New Ortho beds needed for new volume.

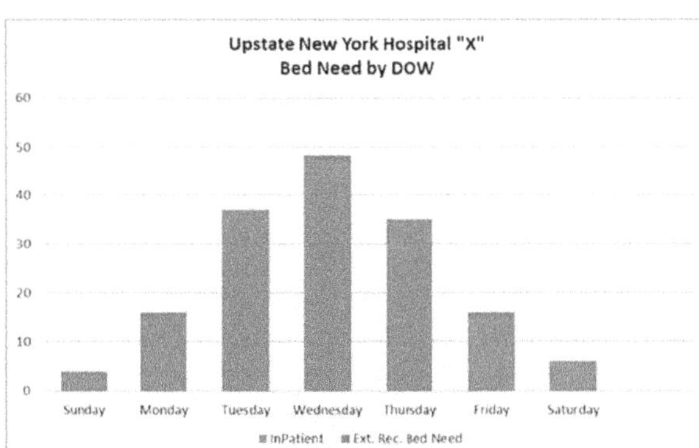

Figure 14.4 Ortho beds need adjusted for extended stay cases.

average lengths of stay for each patient type, a determination of daily inpatient bed need can be made. In the prior graph, the number of orthopedic unit beds needed would be 47 on Wednesday.

The next graph reveals that only 30 beds would be needed if the scheduling process were leveled in relationship to procedure type and length of stay (Figure 14.5).

This leveling process still has significant variability in it because it's being leveled for a 5-day week as shown in the next graph (Figure 14.6).

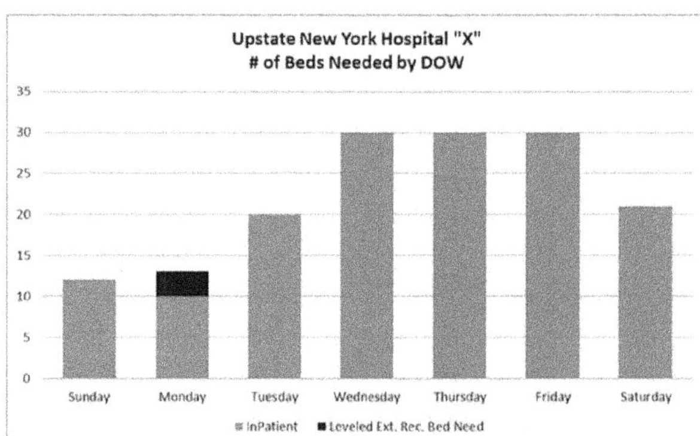

Figure 14.5 Ortho beds needed if Ortho Surgical schedule were leveled.

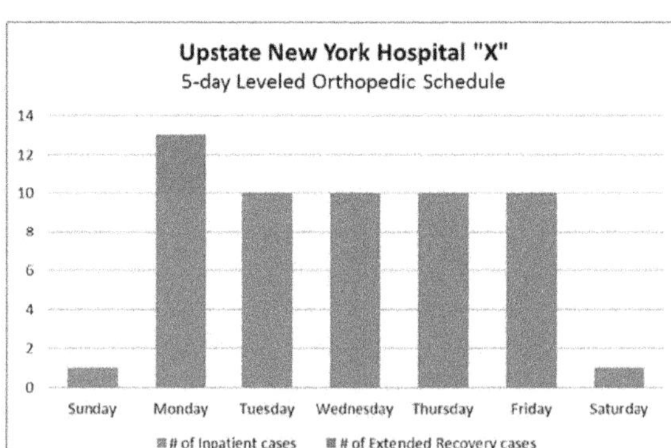

Figure 14.6 Ortho Surgical 5-day leveling.

In its purest form, with 7 days leveled, the number of beds required to manage the patients would drop even further. A 7-day a week Operating Room, correctly leveled, would deliver a number of additional benefits:

(1) Fewer Operating Rooms needed
(2) Lower Operating Room overtime
(3) Fewer patient transfers on and off specialty units for bed needs
(4) Optimal scheduling of ancillary staff such as physical therapy
(5) Leveled transfers to outpatient rehab, be it home or elsewhere

These are just some of the profound secondary impacts that leveling can provide, some of which carry immense financial and logistical benefits to the entire system.

When it becomes clear that a particular process improvement program is not going to be successful (such as leveling), an alternative plan needs to be examined. The following would be considered a short-term alternative to get some improved capacity while trying to determine when to get a leveling program initiated.

Chapter 15

Ancillary Demand Staffing

Current health systems are plagued by bottlenecks and inefficiency. Much time and effort are expended on trying to service multiple components of the health care system and when demand for ancillary services is exceeded, some components will be delayed.

The solution to this has been to look at artificial variability and smooth the variability to improve efficiency and streamline the process, a standard industrial practice. In health care, this model is challenging secondary to:

(1) Political challenges
(2) Financial challenges
(3) Private physician models
(4) Life-style impact related to week-end rounding

These challenges become significant, especially in the surgical realm. Health care is a unique financial model not emulated in the real industrial world and controlled by multiple bodies including governmental agencies, commercial insurers, and other regulatory bodies. This has resulted in a model that is driven predominantly by higher margin surgical cases. When 35% of the admission volume is providing 60% of the revenue, then a mismatch resulting in selective priorities and significant decision-making power by minorities rules the day.

If indeed OR leveling for example is an area which cannot be impacted secondary to reasons given, then organizationally decisions must be made to accommodate this artificial variability. In essence, the OR would be viewed as a variable model BUT with known impact on ancillary demands.

An example would be orthopedic surgery. The current orthopedic schedule is highly variable with 85% plus of cases scheduled on Monday and Tuesday. Standard orthopedic LOS is 3 days and results in the majority of these cases being discharged on Thursday and Friday. This type of scheduling places significant demand on ancillary services. Radiology is now in high demand in the OR on Monday and Tuesday drawing resources away from ED, Floor units, or scheduled outpatients. Physical Therapy is in high demand Tuesday through Friday based on the large volume of orthopedic cases and draws resources away from the floors which may result in delays in discharge or disposition and increase LOS.

Ancillary demand level staffing would provide accommodation for these known variables by adjusting resource allocation to level the needs of all organizationally and improve overall system performance and efficiency. This is an option to at least consider.

Chapter 16

Surge

When hospital capacity is exceeded, SURGE is implemented in order to allow for decompression. This involves the activation of unique processes across the entire hospital. This is *always* an ED phenomenon. I have and likely will never see a hospital on SURGE caused by the OR or Cath Lab schedule. Yet, these units often strain the ED with high scheduled volumes, sometimes increasing the likelihood of SURGE conditions occurring. The outbreak of influenza or a raging GI bug going through the community can also trigger a SURGE response. On rare events, a major traumatic issue can occur with a bus crash or multiple motor vehicle accidents, but almost always the cause is a significant rise in patients presenting to the ED who are deemed in need of hospitalization and beds are unavailable (Table 16.1).

The primary goal in capacity management is to never go on SURGE and always be one step ahead of the need for hospital beds. While designed to accommodate an influx of hospitalizations beyond the hospital's normal operating capacity, SURGE is to be avoided whenever possible because it is expensive, highly stressful on both staff and patients, and is less than ideal for the proper provision of care for every

Table 16.1 Indicators for Hospital Flow and Triggers for SURGE

Indicators of Hospital Flow
Level of Response determined by flow of patients through the Emergency Department and Surgical Department.
Status of the ED is an indicator of patient flow through the House.

- Med/Surg House Census >95%
- Surgical Inpatient Schedule >25% of Total Surgical Beds
- ICU's <3 open beds
- Cath Outpatient Schedule >30% of Cardiac Beds

Triggers for Overcapacity/Surge
- Emergence Department Admit Boarders:

a) 10 boarders; b) 15 boarders; c) 30 boarders; d) >40 boarders
→ each level triggers a flex bed response to bring the Emergence Department back down to a safe manageable level.

patient. Accurate assessment of the status of the hospital at any given point is imperative. Triggers for activation of SURGE must be clear and agreed upon by all. Activation should be in a series of steps and include regular (hourly) assessments of the SURGE status throughout.

Prediction of potential SURGE can be easily accomplished by knowledgeable bed czars. They know the OR and Cath lab schedule, the anticipated discharges for the day, and the hourly admission rate through the ED and will see clear indicators that will result in SURGE activation. Hospitals must first define what the key indicators for activation are and when activation should occur. The when is extremely important since in many high-volume Emergency Departments indicators for SURGE activation can be reached routinely at 3 or 4 pm. The OR's are packed as is the Cath lab, discharges come too late and ED admission volume swells.

The best time we have found for SURGE determination is 8 pm at night. If indicators hit SURGE criteria then, it is highly unlikely that criteria to come off SURGE will occur overnight.

This is because the last discharge leaves the hospital somewhere between 8 pm and 9 pm. Meanwhile, ongoing admissions through the ED will continue to occur (though at a lower rate) all night long. After 8 pm, things are unlikely to improve.

If, at 8 pm, the total hospital bed availability is less than three beds, not including ICUs and ED admissions with unassigned beds and, the overall ED admissions boarding exceeds 30% of ED adult bed capacity, then SURGE is activated. One issue that occurs with a late activation is that holding personnel longer or extending testing hours will be difficult to achieve since most of these individuals have left for the day. A compromise is to have necessary personnel start the next day earlier if the hospital is still in surge mode.

Once these criteria have been reached, communication must occur to a broad group of individuals. A domino effect is intended, activating non-clinical space and providing extended service capability in a step-by-step process. It is important to note that SURGE does not change organizational priorities—its purpose is to allow the overall system to continue to manage patients entering the system from all portals of entry---ED, OR, Cath lab and directs and transfers, and to ease the overburdened ED.

A Surge team membership is well established in advance. A typical Surge team would include ED Director, Hospitalist director, Bed-management director, Cath lab director, OR/PACU director, Administrative representative, med/surg floor director, Radiology director, and Echo/Stress test director.

A typical Surge process, organized into steps, is as follows:

Step-1. A text message is sent to SURGE team members to notify of SURGE activation.

Step-2. Environmental services set up hall-way beds in various med/surg units to flex capacity—this is typically 1–2 beds per unit.

Step-3. A 7 am team meeting for 5 min determines the anticipated bed needs for the day based on the current state of the ED, OR and Cath lab schedules, expected incoming transfers, and expected discharge volume. This short meeting will also determine what flex space beyond the anticipated hallway beds will be utilized.

Step-4. Determine Flex space to be used, such as Cath Lab holding, Boarding in PACU, and other identified hospital space suitable for patients. These may vary by institution and availability, but the Surge team must all be clear on a specific plan, which should be put into action immediately. PACU holds, for example, should focus on patients who are considered extended recovery cases and have a high likelihood of discharge the next morning.

Step-5. Extended Service Capability—Testing hours are extended. These usually involve Cardiac studies, nuclear stress tests, Echos, MRIs, CTs, USN, and other stress testing and Radiographic studies. The facilities and staff that normally would operate with limited hours will now need to implement extended hours to provide testing to all patients whose disposition status and potential discharge may be dependent on them. All disposition studies should be completed on all hospitalized patients by extending these service hours, including the reading of these studies. Consideration should be made to prioritize inpatient testing over scheduled outpatients. If it is felt to be a need to initiate availability of certain study types early in the am, that decision should be directed to the appropriate study area at step 2.

Step-6. Focus on discharges. Hospitalists should focus efforts on early discharges while environmental services focus on immediate room cleans and communication back to bed assignment. Administrative representation is to concur and validate the need for overtime services and additional staff if necessary.

Step-7. Hourly assessment—The criteria to remain in SURGE and to continue to utilize alternative clinical space and extended service hours is conducted hourly. Team members should reconvene at appropriate intervals, usually around noon and 4 pm, to determine challenges and utilization of other strategies if necessary. Maintaining use of non-clinical space for patients such as hallways, Cath-lab holding areas, or the PACU in OR recovery need to be taken into account for additional staffing resources if required.

Only when the system has decompressed below the initiating SURGE criteria should SURGE activation be canceled. Debriefs should occur with the team to determine if all components were activated as anticipated and what could be done in the future to avert SURGE activation or once initiated to cancel SURGE activation as quickly as possible.

Chapter 17

Starting a Patient Flow Team

So, you've been called into the Hospitals CEO's office and told to develop a Patient Flow Team. You could be a Physician, Nurse Leader, Administrator, or other individual in the hospital's leadership lineup. Where do you start? Who do you ask to join and what are you expected to do? Having been down this road, I will offer some advice and strategies to assist in the implementation of a Patient Flow team.

The first thing to understand is that hospitals function very much like industry. Yes. I have heard all the quotes like, "we're not making camera's here buddy," or "we aren't building cars here." In reality, there are significant similarities between industry and healthcare. Both are trying to achieve the most efficient way to produce a product, be that a car or a healthy patient. See the figure below.

You can see in Figure 17.1 that in the Healthcare arena that the industrial process has been mirrored. You will also notice that there are two equal signs and the words hard and easy below the captions. These give you an idea of the complexity of evaluating and managing each component. So, patient transport from point A to B is considered the easiest. Equally

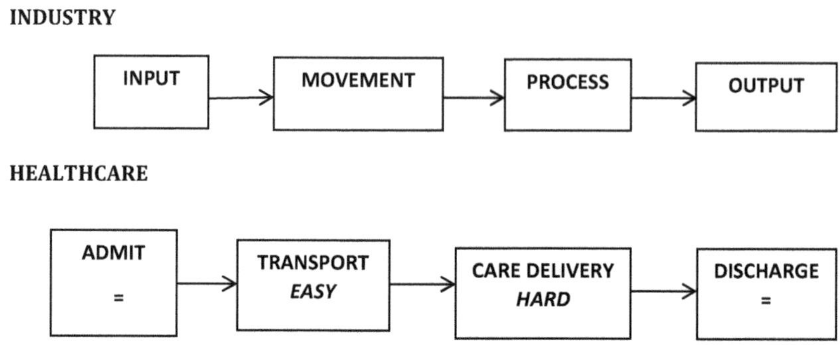

Figure 17.1 Industry workflow versus healthcare workflow.

difficult are the admission process and the discharge process. The most complex to undertake is the care delivery process because of the multitude of factors that must be taken into account. So where do you start? The first order of business is to develop what I refer to as a steering committee. This is a group of high-level leaders that determine what projects will have the highest priority and report results to the executive C-suite. The components of the steering committee might include:

(1) Physician
(2) Nurse
(3) Bed Assignment
(4) Transport
(5) Environmental Services
(6) Social Work
(7) Care Management
(8) Administration
(9) Ancillary—IT, Pharmacy, Lab, Radiology, Specialty Consults-PT, Respiratory, Nutrition, etc.

Experience taught me that just because individuals reach a high level of leadership in a healthcare organization, it does not necessarily correlate with getting things done. The result was the development of a team we called the "TENS" committee. So, what is the "TENS" committee? Individuals in the hospital know the people who can get things done if given the opportunity and the authority to work freely and creatively. These are the "TENS" of the organization. This is a small committee made up of perhaps five hand selected individuals to implement project change. It could be a nurse manager, or a Hospitalist or someone from Bed Assignment, or perhaps a high functioning Transporter or Environmental service member. You would be surprised about the importance in any hospital project of Bed Assignment, Transport, and Environmental Services.

Once you have your committee members selected, they will all need focus on what metrics they are going to try an impact. These metrics need to be agreed upon by the members and they have to be readily available, valid, and reported out in a timely fashion.

An example of focused metrics is the table below (Table 17.1):

Your group may have a different focus, and this is just an example. I would like to point out that each of these metrics aligns with one of the four components we previously described—Admit (ED Hold Time & 30-day readmits)—Transport (ED Hold Time)—Care Delivery (LOS & Patient Satisfaction)—Discharge (Discharge before noon & 30-day readmit).

Table 17.1 Focused Metrics Decided upon by Steering Group of the "Flow Team." Metrics Followed Daily Then Reported Weekly and Monthly. Shared Universally, and Used to Indicate Achievements and Where More Attention Is Needed

Metric	*Goal*	*Result*
LOS	4.5 days	
D/C before noon	30%	
30 Day Readmit	10%	
ED Hold Time	240 minutes	
Patient Satisfaction	80th percentile	

So now you have your team members identified and your focused metrics. The next step is to determine frequency of meeting times. We found that in order to keep things moving aggressively, weekly meetings worked best. One key point about these meetings. In healthcare, leadership usually has a number of meetings that are scheduled daily. These meetings will have priorities either identified by the leadership or the individual. Meetings which individuals do not enjoy attending for whatever reason can become low on the priority list and no one shows up at the weekly meeting with multiple reasons why. It should be made clear by leadership that this is a priority for the organization and as such these are priority meetings that are to be attended weekly unless individuals are absent from the organization.

Now that you have your members, meeting frequency, and focused metrics, the next step is to determine what to do. Where do you focus your energy? What projects give you the biggest bang for the buck? Is the issue ED boarders, problematic discharge, increased length of stay? I have put together a 4-phase operational strategy that organizations can follow in improving overall patient flow. The phases are designed to first make sure the hospital is getting paid for what they are doing, are compliant, and develop a good understanding of baseline data elements.

The second phase deals predominantly with hospital operational metrics with a primary focus on the “Patient Flow” metrics dashboard outlined previously.

The third phase deals with process redesign. The nitty gritty of understanding how things currently work and how care is delivered. This is the heart of the Patient Flow team focus.

The last phase deals with complex process design. This takes on the challenging areas of leveling, demand level staffing and space utilization.

Depending where your organization currently is regarding process improvement and redesign, you can determine what phase you should focus on. There are some key factors that need to always be taken into account.

(1) Proactive management of the hospital is necessary to achieve success.
(2) Changes in Culture (Behavior) are predominantly done through influence and diplomacy.
(3) Communication is essential. The more the better. Everyone needs to know what you're doing and why, how you're doing from a measurement perspective and what areas are being focused on for improvement.
(4) DATA-DATA-DATA It must be available, accurate, timely, and easily understood.
(5) Last—It is all about the PATIENT. A well-run efficient hospital will achieve lower unexpected outcomes, higher patient satisfaction, greater employee satisfaction, and be financially successful.

Chapter 18

Optimal Hospital Operational Strategies

Phase I

Strategies in phase I surround functional and operational design of the hospital to maximize bed utilization and develop an intake and output model that manages regulatory compliance. This phase is divided into four primary components.

Medical Necessity: This component is mandatory for accurate patient classification, compliance, billing, and denials management. Hospital entry points for medical necessity are as follows.

Emergency Department Admissions—divided into Inpatient or Observation status
Cath lab procedures—divided into inpatient or outpatient
Operating Room procedures—divided into Outpatient, 23 Hour extended Recovery (still outpatient) and Inpatient.

The main purpose of these classifications is related to acuity of illness utilizing InterQual guidelines as a basis for the initial classification. These classes have significance in determining a hospital's level of compliance set forth by the government and also establish a level of organizational confidence in defense of medical necessity determinations for commercial insurers. Significant swings in percentage of patient classification can lead to profound changes in revenue predications and strategies surrounding hospital bed modeling.

The primary determination of level of care (medical necessity) is performed by physicians in conjunction with "Care Management." Since determinations must be made at the time of admission to the hospital, care management plays a critical role in evaluating both the primary determination and ongoing determinations of medical necessity during a patient's hospitalization.

Optimal design will be dependent on volume of cases and case mix, but strategies need to deploy care management in four primary locations or be linked to them to be effective.

Those locations are:

Emergency Department
Cath Lab
Post-Operative Care Area
Med/Surg Floors

The three primary entry points, and design elements, are for initial determination levels of medical necessity and the med/surg component is necessary for re-evaluation of patients when medical necessity reviews result in a change of patient classification.

Centralized Bed Assignment

Maximal bed utilization can only be obtained by centralizing the responsibilities for the placement of patients in hospital beds. Centralized bed assignment is effective only when the hospital operational model has developed a set of priorities surrounding bed utilization and patient placement. These priorities must be followed and understood by all hospital departments.

Bed Assignment Priority

ICU bed availability—Sickest First
Operating Room Patients
Cath Lab Patients
Directs or Transfers

Emergency Department Admissions

Maintaining these priorities allows centralized bed management to make strategic decisions which impact care delivery, optimal bed utilization, and priority placement of patients requiring hospital beds. Use of "Bed Ahead" strategies can be beneficial to maintaining the hospitals ability to serve its patients and use resources in the most efficient manner. Proactive techniques including "Next Week" planning and holding beds in specialty areas of the hospital on Sunday nights can be effective in limiting movement of patients from one unit to another to maintain this priority-based structure.

Hospital Bed Construct

To effectively implement strategies surrounding hospital operational modeling, the hospital bed construct must be designed to consider both the types of patients seen, the service components the hospital has in place, and the growth and vision of hospital management. Hospital bed construct can be divided into the following categories:

Licensed Hospital beds—those beds built and approved for use by patients requiring hospital admission and include ICU beds and med/surg beds

Unlicensed hospital beds—include areas in which patients are housed but do not exist on the hospitals unlicensed bed list: Emergency Department, PACU, Cath lab holding, Observation units, and hallway beds.

Although bed type and utilization may be directed by government regulation, the ability to identify the hospital's needs and develop a bed construct around those needs will significantly impact overall efficiency and flow of patients through the organization. Med/surg beds can be considered under two primary categories:

Specialty beds—Orthopedic, Stroke, Cardiac, etc.
Generic beds—Any patient may utilize the bed

Limitations of the generic bed construct are usually centered around hospital bed numbers and acuity of illness. As hospital services broaden and the acuity of illness increases, specialty utilization becomes a more specific model.

The primary design of bed construct determines needs for acuity, how best to cluster patient types to gain efficiency of care delivery and measure impact on hospital Length of Stay, and other metrics which determine both the quality and operational effectiveness of the organization. An example is Observation Beds—Since this patient type is designated as outpatient, any bed in the hospital can be a recipient of this patient type. This includes Emergency Room beds, Observation Unit Specific beds and med/surg beds. The impact of this variable bed use has implications surrounding efficiency of patient movement and cost of patient care. Using ED beds for observation uses highly skilled staff to manage lower-level acuity patients and impacts Emergency Bed availability during high census resulting in potential delays in new patient evaluations, increased left without being seen rates, and hospital diversion of EMS.

Use of med/surg beds in a scatter-bed arrangement for observation type patients results in increased LOS, lack of focus on lower acuity patients, and improved bed turns.

Clearly the hospital size, acuity, and occupancy rates would drive hospital construct in a specific direction. Lack of clustering specific patient types (observation and outpatient surgery) regardless of hospital size will not allow the organization to take advantage of the efficient impact this strategy can have on bed utilization and LOS.

Denials Management

Denials management from a system's perspective links to medical necessity and the development of a system which accurately identifies level of care, upgrades that level from an outpatient to an inpatient status when identified, and can effectively defend the organizations decisions when questioned by either governmental agencies or commercial insurers. Denials fall into three primary areas:

1. Medical necessity denials-or level of care—these may also include denials of bed days based on documented patient acuity
2. HIM denials—primarily DRG designations which are directed by provider documentation
3. Billing denials—these are usually clerical denials in the form of incorrect demographics or other incorrect billing components.

The use of a denials management system for the hospital requires a centralized area for denials which then filter and dispense the denials into those areas which have the proper expertise and team members to effectively manage the denials. The need for Physician oversight cannot be underestimated. Both the medical necessity and HIM denials can clearly be filtered by Utilization management personnel, but physician leadership is mandatory. This construct will allow the most effective focus on denials and can monitor areas requiring operational improvement on the front-end process of medical necessity. With constant monitoring and effective management, the impact on reduction in denials by both governmental agencies and commercial insures will have significant impact on organizational finances and resources required to manage this process.

Phase II

Operational metrics to establish quality indicators, organizational effectiveness, monitoring of process improvement activities, and compliance of governmental standards must be established to provide organizational focus on resource allocation and establishment of organizational strategies.

System metrics are necessary to establish baseline practice and must be valid and acquired from a single reliable source. Hospital metrics from a system perspective need to have an ability to drill down to the individual provider level to determine areas of opportunity for improvement. The following metrics are a guide to operational efficiency:

Hospital length of stay preference would be in hours
Discharges before noon
30-day readmissions
Patient satisfaction

Each of these components link to quality, efficiency, finance, and service. Additional metrics used for operational assessment include:

Governmental Metrics: This includes core measures, reports on hospital utilization, Program for Evaluating Payment Patterns Electronic Report (PEPPER), Hospital Consumer Assessment of Healthcare Providers and Systems(HCHAPS) hospital acquired infections, and others

Quality Metrics: Includes "never" events, hospital errors-meds, blood draws, wrong patient studies, falls, and others

Financial Metrics: Days cash on hand, debt level, collection rates, bad debt, and others

Efficiency Metrics: Includes patient movement—ED to admit time, admit to bed placement time, ED to ICU transfer time, PACU to floor time, and others

The importance of a centralized storehouse of metrics is mandatory. As drill downs occur and departments develop effective methods to gauge their efficiency, linkage must be maintained to the overall system metrics which determine optimal operational efficiency.

Phase III: Process Redesign

Process redesign brings focus and resources to areas of opportunity defined by metrics. Areas of opportunity may be defined by comparisons to similar organizations, best practice, or complete redesign strategies using industry accepted methodologies and include:

An organizational and operational effectiveness assessment using Lean Six-Sigma methodologies

The development of an efficiency improvement plan that aligns with the organizations strategic needs and design elements specified in phase I.

The design and structuring of a process improvement strategy includes the following:

An internal training and capability development plan for process improvement (Lean Sigma) expertise

The development of standards and escalation processes to ensure sustainment of improvements

The development of standard work for leadership at all levels: This supports their role in leading through the use of continuous improvement methodologies and processes (Lean Sigma)

A financial improvement plan based on the tactical deployment of Lean Sigma methodologies targeting patient flow and throughput improvements

Process Redesign has multiple components to it. Primary areas of focus would be as follows:

Non-Care Delivery Process improvement: Primary focus is on accuracy of non-clinical components which begin at the point of patient registration and end at the point of clean claims billing. This includes evaluation using Lean to look at the entire non-patient care delivery process and would evolve:

Patient Access and Registration
Clinical Documentation (provider)
Enhanced Clinical Documentation Review and Education
Optimal Coding and Educational Formats
Optimal Billing with high percentages of Clean Claims and minimal discharge to dropped bill days
Impact of process on denials management

Material and Supplies

This area has significant opportunity especially under management of inventory and use, standardization of product, contract management of vendors, and maintaining best practice standards in the organization. High use areas would be the primary focus and would include:

Operating Rooms
Cath Labs
Emergency Services
Pharmacy
ICUs

Patient Care Delivery

Process Redesign begins with care delivery. The design must have two guiding principles:

(1) Patient Centered
(2) Error Free

The patient care delivery process improvement models focus need to be at the front end and requires optimal completion of components required to process patient admissions. These components include:

Physician
Nurse
APP-NP or PA
Pharmacist

Process improvement results in immediate institution of care delivery with timely administration of medications for the patient's acute needs but also addresses the patient's needs for medications used for chronic conditions. Medication reconciliation can be completed promptly and correctly. A complete head to toe nursing assessment is completed and eliminates duplication on the med/surg floors.

The second component is the patient movement in a timely fashion to the area of the hospital that can best serve the patient's needs. This process needs to adhere to organizational priorities and would include focus on:

ED to ICU transfers (sickest first philosophy)
ED to OR transfers
ED to Floor Transfers

Operational metrics would drive the process improvement to provide ED patients to exit to the proper care delivery area in a timely fashion once a bed has been acquired.

The third component is the care delivery provided on the hospital units. The concept of team-based care needs to be understood and will be most successful if a geographic model is utilized to allow staffing of team members to maintain availability on the unit where care is being delivered. Construct of a geographic model may vary from one institution to another but the primary focus of managing rooms which contain a patient with a team is most important. This provides multiple positive impacts including precise and consistent communication, timely interventions, and a non-silo approach to care delivery.

The last process is one of consistent and standard discharge plans which will communicate to the patient any changes in the management of their disease, communicate with the follow-up physician or facility and the effectiveness is measured with metrics that are defined as key to organizational success—30-day readmissions, discharges before noon, and patient satisfaction.

Ancillary Care Delivery Redesign

The components which impact care delivery are many times ancillary in nature and may impact all or a subset of patients cared for. These components are:

Lab
Radiology
Pharmacy
Cardiac Testing
Non-Provider Consults-PT, OT, nutritional
Provider Consults-GI, Cards, ENT, etc.

Each should have standard benchmarks for providing defined service to patients being cared for. The use of Lean in their evaluation is of utmost importance.

Phase IV: Complex Process Redesign

The components of this phase require the organization to have reached a mature level of managing change and utilizing Lean to improve the organizational efficiency. The components to focus on for complex design will have significant financial impact surrounding demand level staffing, space utilization, and leveling. The areas of focus would be as follows:

Demand Level Staffing

ED
Cath Lab
Operating Room
Clinics
Inpatient Providers Staffing

Space Utilization

ED
Cath Lab Rooms
Operating Rooms
Other procedural rooms

Leveling (Elective Scheduling)

Cath Lab Schedule
Operating Schedule
Other elective schedule

These complex processes will require significant resources and clearly defined metrics to monitor success. Profound changes in behavior and current processes will be required to achieve the impact that these areas could have on operational efficiency and costs.

Chapter 19

Process Improvement

There are many ideas, often competing with one another, for improving our healthcare system. There are also many pressures bearing on every healthcare administration, each pushing or pulling its decision-making process in different directions. New laws, such as Obamacare, government oversight, penalties, complex billing systems, shifting and nebulous rules and regulations, insurance interests, competition, financial strains, competing interests within the hospital community, and many other factors come in to play. And at the center of it all, hopefully, is the drive to deliver world-class care to patients.

But when an administration weighs every argument and option, how should it act? Many hospitals make a decision to improve some process or other or reorganize itself for efficiency or for better care outcomes, only to fail once the carefully championed, budgeted, and managed project hits the hospital floor. Hospital processes, people, and infrastructure are notoriously entrenched and difficult to reform. When starting this improvement journey, the system must not go at this haphazardly. The improvement methodologies should be structured and consistent throughout the healthcare organization. Methodologies can be singular or blended, that is, Six Sigma, Lean, Lean Six Sigma. Oft times when either of these are used by themselves, changes are not sustainable, resulting in the expenditure of resources without return and Leadership and front-line staff are left with a bad taste in their mouths toward Change.

The methodology we have found to result in sustainable change is Lean Six Sigma. This methodology is based not only on data but includes buy-in and involvement of front-line staff and Leadership all the way up to the CEO. This involvement results in ownership of the change by both front-line team members and those leading the system. The tools of Lean are easily taught and used by System Leaders and Front Line. When plans for change are developed and implemented by Front Line there is a greater chance for sustainability. The advantage of combining Lean Methodologies with Six-Sigma is timeliness and speed. Where projects using only Six-Sigma methodologies may take upward to 6–12 months to put a pilot in place, the addition of Lean results in analysis, piloting, and implementing change in as short a time as 4–6 weeks.

This book has focused on the Hospital Emergency Department and related units. Our ideas are those that we know, we have put many of them into practice, or otherwise been involved in their development. The ideas in this book are mostly all tested, in that they have been put into practice in hospitals and have been shown to be successful for the most part. We have witnessed both success and failure in this realm and have learned that the two outcomes are often separated by the thinnest of margins. Hospitals that consider and address the following points will be far more likely to succeed in any initiative than those that fail to do so. Just look at today's prevalence of scatter-bed observation units. There is little evidence to suggest that this approach is better, either for patients or for the hospital. But it is the way we have always done things.

Therefore, we would advise that any administration considering any of our recommended initiatives, or any other for that matter, should first ensure that the following considerations are discussed and dealt with. In our experience, failure to do so can jeopardize success. Any project, in order to succeed, must consider the following:

Project Focus: Everyone must understand the goal of the project. What is the driving force behind it? It must have at its center the care of the patient. Will it impact strategic metrics for the organization? Is it aligned with organizational priorities? There should be no questions left standing before any project can be expected to succeed.

Data: Getting accurate baseline data is absolutely essential to any process improvement. Understanding the current metric that you wish to impact and having the ability to obtain that metric in a consistent and valid fashion is of utmost importance. Without this information, the project's value will be unknown, its faults will potentially go unnoticed, rather than being quickly spotted and addressed, and its detractors will go unanswered.

Leadership: Developing a team of people to manage the project is crucial. The optimal team size is around five people. Team members may have sub-teams, but the leadership needs to be small and focused. Success generally only occurs if one high level C-suite member is driving meetings and holding all team members accountable for results. Countless projects fall victim to poor communication, distraction, mission fatigue, and lack of accountability, all of which is addressed with a strong leadership team.

Timeline: Further focus on leadership and accountability is a solid timeline that helps keep a project on track. There should be a published schedule for meetings, along with monitoring of baseline metrics such as, current process analysis, development of improved process redesign and implementation and monitoring of the process redesigned. Project completion times will vary, but many in our experience take around 6 months depending on the project's complexity.

Scaling: Organizations tend to want projects implemented system wide and usually in very short time frames. But complex processes within healthcare take time to reinvent and implement—and sometimes require a bit of tinkering in practice. Many successful projects use a single unit as a guinea pig, of sorts, working out bugs and establishing best practices first. Then, the project can more easily be scaled to other units, eventually achieving the goal of overall sustainable organizational change, but with less risk of an overall organizational failure.

Celebration: It will take a great deal of hard work and dedication to achieve success—and it's important that everyone involved is recognized for their effort, especially when a project has proven to be successful. This is not only a boost for morale and good publicity for a success but helps encourage participation and expectations of success for future projects.

Below are two examples of actual projects that we have been involved with. Both projects are highly typical of almost any hospital system's effort to improve, and both could have easily failed (one certainly did). But they are both good examples of what can go wrong and right in any project.

ED to ICU Transfer Project

Project Focus

Improve ICU mortality rate: This particular project was brought about after two ICU mortality cases were analyzed. It was found that delays between the ED and transfer to the ICU were the primary cause of death. This conclusion was also supported by medical literature, which closely correlates mortality of ICU patients with length of stay in the ED.

Data

The baseline time for a patient to get to the ICU once admitted in the ED was 6 h on average. I distinctly remember one of our first meetings when the discussion turned to our goal. We had discussed cutting it in half, then to 2 h. Finally, I mentioned that we really already had a process of getting patients requiring the ICU out of the ED in less than 60 min. Everyone stared. The Door to Balloon time for acute MI patients presenting to the ED was rapidly approaching the 60-min mark. Whether someone is septic or having an acute myocardial infarction, their transfer time should be no different. So, 60 min was determined to be the benchmark we would shoot for.

Leadership

Our team was the following: ICU representative, ED representative, Bed assignment, Hospitalist representative, Administrative representative.

Timeline

Our team determined we would need 6 months to complete the project.

Scaling

The project was limited to a single process transferring from ED to ICU—no scaling needed to be considered.

With a plan in mind, our team first set out to determine what the current process was for identifying and then transferring an ICU patient from the ED. It was extremely complex. We found that depending on the time of day, there were different phone calls to make, and that, further complicating things, there were different people responsible for determining whether the patient should go to the ICU. We also found that perceptions had developed that the ED was placing patients in the ICU just to get them out of the ED. Also, there was no electronic method to track data. We mapped out the whole convoluted process and quickly the whole team understood that we needed a streamlined process, with only one phone call to make and a mechanism to track progress.

The concept of using an identified ICU nurse as the focal point of communication was developed. This person had two primary responsibilities:

(1) Initiate the cascade of events that needed to occur when called for with a patient requiring ICU care
(2) Always have an ICU bed available for the next ICU patient

This person would also fill out the hand log to track the patients and metrics.

The new process was implemented but not without problems. Everyday follow-up phone calls would be made to providers involved with any ICU patient whose transfer process exceeded our benchmark. Weeks went by and slowly we got consistently below the 2-h mark. Then months later, we gradually began to achieve the 60-min mark. This is a critical point in projects. Too often, hospitals achieve results and then move on to other things. The project was handed over to the hospitalist group. We watched as the numbers started getting right back to baseline. The team looked at what was happening and concluded that the provider follow-up was no longer there. We had learned that it was integral to the process.

The project was then handed to the physician director of the ICU who truly took ownership. They got the project back on track and to this day, it remains a significant success.

Celebration

Two interesting downstream effects came out of this project. Raw mortality for ICU patients dropped an astonishing 15% and the length of stay of ICU patients dropped by almost a day. In hospital capacity management, these are the kinds of projects and successes you live for. Some of us still celebrate the success to this day.

Reduction in Operating Room Turn Times

Project Focus

The concern was that the volume of scheduled operations was more than the Operating Rooms could handle. Our goal was to reduce Operating Room turnaround times, effectively boosting available room time to handle demand.

Data

Operating Room start times were dismal. Average delays were around 12 min. In a unique move, the room set-up process was videotaped and reviewed. This revealed that 8 min could be saved, only by removing redundancies in the work process. We believed that with minor impact, and some training, we could save 20 min between each case. This may not sound like a great deal, but when we calculated daily savings over the current system, it came to a whopping 500 min each day. This is the equivalent of freeing up an entire Operating Room. It costs 5 million dollars to build an Operating Room, and another $1,000 an hour to run it. Our study had revealed a very significant cost saving.

Leadership

Our team was the following: OR representative, Administrative representative, PACU representative, Bed Assignment, and Lean Sigma representative

Timeline

Out Team determined we would need 2 months to conclude study.

Scaling

If we could find any savings in one room, it could be scaled to every OR in the system.

After our analysis and conclusions were complete, the recommendations were presented. Everyone agreed that the recommendations, if acted upon, would save the system millions of dollars, with very little upfront cost. Success would be highly likely. But the result was not success. No one was willing to hold surgeons accountable for on-time starts. There is little will within many hospitals to fight this kind of fight, and in this particular case, the project was shelved and put on hold indefinitely.

The lesson here is that accountability is key to managing changes in health care. There is significant reluctance, however, to hold senior physicians to account, or to demand that they change their schedules, lifestyles, expectations, or habits in any way. To do so is very uncomfortable and takes a great deal of effort. Ultimately, it may take a reminder that accountability for patient care rests on those physician's shoulders, and that sometimes a change of habit or a coveted tee-off time is simply the right thing to do. Again, we must keep the patient at the center of our healthcare system.

Chapter 20

Conclusion

I do hope you have enjoyed this book on managing hospital capacity. The focus is really on the patient. A well-run hospital incorporating components within this book will be light years ahead in the healthcare delivery of patients. I suspect that slowly over the next 30 or 40 years, a number of these processes will be implemented in some way, shape, or form in our Healthcare system. There is currently a major focus on patient flow and patient safety within hospitals. I would encourage more investment in capacity management because the impacts of it will result in a much safer experience for the patient and a much more efficient system to move the patient through the complexities of the healthcare system.

I hope this book becomes your roadmap in hospital capacity management improvement and provides your patients and your organization great success in the future. Thanks for your interest and your time.

Bibliography

1. Kumar, K. et al., How Advanced Analytics Can Improve Hospital Capacity Management, Infosys, 2009, 1–2.
2. Theodore Eugene Day et al., Decreased Length of Stay after Addition of Healthcare Provider in Emergency Department Triage, *Emergency Medicine Journal*, 2013, 30(2), 134–138, bedside registration.
3. Takakuw, K.M. et al., Strategies for Dealing with Emergency Department Overcrowding: A One-Year Study on How Bedside Registration Affects Patient Throughput Times, *The Journal of Emergency Medicine*, 2007, 32, 4, 337–342.
4. Welch, S., In the Zone: Redesigning Flow, *Emergency Medicine News*, 2009, 31(7), 1–4.
5. Chalfin, D. et al., Impact of Delayed Transfer of Critically Ill Patients from the Emergency Department to the Intensive Care Unit, *Critical Care Medicine*, 2007, 35(6), 1477–1483.
6. Macario, A. et al., Anesthesia & Analgesia: Hospital Profitability per Hour of Operating Room Time Can Vary among Surgeons, Sept 2001, 93(3), 669–675.
7. Ryckman, F.C. et al., Cincinnati Children's Hospital Medical Center: Redesigning Perioperative Flow Using Operations Management Tools to Improve Access and Safety: Managing Patient Flow in Hospitals, 2nd ed, Eugene Litvak (ed.), 97–111.
8. Guarisco, J., FAAEM: Fixing the Crowded ED Part 1-Building a Burning Platform, *Medscape*, 2013.
9. Pham, J.C. et al., ACAD EMERG MED: The Effects of Ambulance Diversion: A Comprehensive Review, Nov 2006, 13(11), 1220–1227.

10. *Health Services Cost Review Commission*, Staff Final Recommendations Regarding Medicare's Two Midnight Rule Effective Oct 1, 2013. Health Services Cost Review Commission, 2013, 1–6.
11. Medicare Claims Processing Manual Chapter 1, 50.3.2, Policy and Billing Instructions for Condition Code 44. (Rev 2016, issued: 10-01-10, Effective: 10-01-10, Implementation: 10-04-10).
12. *Interqual-McKesson Health Solutions LLC*, 2020, WWW.Mckesson.com.
13. *Millimans and Roberts, Milliman Care Guidelines, LLC*, 2020 WWW.millimans.com.
14. Nguyen, J.M. et al.. A Universal Method for Determining Intensive Care Unit Bed Requirements, *Intensive Care Medicine*. May 2003, 29(5), 849–852.
15. Renee M. Gindi, Robin A. Cohen, and Whitney K. Kirzinger, January–June 2011, Emergency Room Use Among Adults Aged 18-64: Early Release of Estimates From the National Health Interview Survey, , Division of Health Interview Statistics, National Center for Health Statistics. 5/2012, pages 1–11.
16. Pena, M.E. et al., Effect on Efficiency and Cost-Effectiveness When an Observation Unit is Managed as a Closed Unit vs an Open Unit, *American Journal of Emergency Medicine*, 2013, 31(7), 1042–1046.
17. *Clinical Advisory Board*, 2009, Next Generation Capacity Management, Volume 1, Clinical Advisory Board, Index of Efficiency Metrics, pages 56–57.
18. White, H.L. and Glazier, R.H., Do Hospitalist Physicians Improve the Quality of Inpatient Care Delivery? A Systematic Review of Process, Efficiency and Outcome Measures, *BMC Medicine*, 2011, 9(58), 1–14.
19. Schuur, J.D., The Growing Role of Emergency Departments in Hospital Admissions, *New England Journal of Medicine*, 2012, 367, 391–393.
20. David, J.Y., May 2013, Getting Started: Moving Toward Unit-Based CareTodays Hospitalist, 1–4.
21. Kumar, D. et al., Diagnosis and Timing of 30-Day Readmissions After Hospitalization for Heart Failure, Acute Myocardial Infarction or Pneumonia, 23/30, *JAMA*, 2013, 309, 4.

22. Sara Rosenbaum, J.D., The Patient Protection and Affordable Care Act: Implications for Public Health Policy and Practice, *Public Health Reports*, 2011, 126(1), 130–135.
23. Hanse, L.O. et al., Interventions to Reduce 30-Day Rehospitalization: A Systematic Review, *Annals of Internal Medicine*, 2011, 155(8), 520–528.
24. Beresford, L., Sept 2013, Project BOOST Study Documents Modest Impact on 30-Day Hospital Readmissions, The Hospitalist, 1-3.
25. Coleman, E. et al., Preparing Patients and Caregivers to Participate in Care Delivered Across Settings: The Care Transitions Intervention, *Journal of the American Geriatrics Society*, 52(11), 1817–1825.
26. Jack, B.W. et al., A Reengineered Hospital Discharge Program to Decrease Rehospitalization, *Annals of Internal Medicine*, 2009, 150, 178–187.
27. Boutwell, G.A. et al., *Effective Interventions to Reduce Rehospitalizations: A compendium of 15 Promising Interventions* Cambridge, MA: Institute for Healthcare Improvement, 2009.
28. Berwick, D.M., Nolan, T., and Whittington, J., The Triple Aim: Care, Health, and Cost, *Health Affairs*, 2008, 27(3), 759–769.
29. Churpek, M.M., Wendlandt, B., Zadravecz, F.J., Adhikari, R., Winslow, C., and Edelson, D.P., Association between Intensive Care Unit Transfer Delay and Hospital Mortality: A Multicenter Investigation, *Journal of Hospital Medicine*, 2016, 11, 757–762. doi:10.1002/jhm.2630.
30. Newman, J.S., 2011. Top 10 Reasons Not to Discharge Your Patient. ACP Hospitalist. http://www.acphospitalist.org/archives/2011/09/newman.htm.
31. Kohn, L.T., Corrigan, J., and Donaldson, M.S., 2000, *To Err is Human: Building a Safer Health System*. Washington, DC: National Academy Press.
32. Stein, J., Murphy, D., and Payne, C., A Remedy for Fragmented Healthcare, *Harvard Business Review*, 2013. Retrieved January 7, 2015, from https://hbr.org/2013/11/a-remedy-for-fragmented-hospital-care.
33. Jack, B.W., Chetty, V.K., Anthony, D., Greenwald, J.L., Sanchez, G.M., Johnson, A.E. et al., A Reengineered Hospital Discharge Program to Decrease Rehospitalization: A Randomized

Trial, *Annals of Internal Medicine*, 2009, 150, 178–187. doi: 10.7326/0003-4819-150-3-200902030-00007.

34. O'Reilly, K.B., February 18, 2013, AMA Details Plan for Cutting Hospital Readmissions. Retrieved from http://www.amednews.com/article/20130218/health/130219952/4/.
35. O'Leary, K.J., Kulkarni, N., Landler, M. P., Jeon, J., Hahn, K.J., Englert, K.M., and Williams, M.V., Hospitalized Patients' Understanding of Their Plan of Care, *Mayo Clinic Proceedings*, 2010, *85*(1), 47–52. 10.4065/mcp.2009.0232.
36. Baugh, C.W., Liang, L.J., and Sun, B.C., 9 National Cost Savings from Observation Unit of Management of Syncope,*Annals of Emergency Medicine,* 2014, *64*(4), S15.
37. Khare, R.K., Powell, E.S., Reinhardt, G., and Lucenti, M., Adding More Beds to the Emergency Department or Reducing Admitted Patient Boarding Times: Which Has a More Significant Influence on Emergency Department Congestion?, *Annals of Emergency Medicine,* 2009, 575–585. 10.1016/j.annemergmed.2008.07.009.
38. *Joint Commission Perspectives*, Standards Revisions Addressing Patient Flow through the Emergency Department, Volume 32, Issue 7, July 2012, 1–5.
39. Keith D. Hentel et al., What Physicians and Health Organizations Should Know About Mandated Imaging Appropriate Use Criteria, *Annals of Internal Medicine,* June 2019, 170, 12–18, 880-885.
40. Daly, M.L., Powers, J., and Orto, V., Early Nursing Intervention Beyond Rapid Response Teams, Institute for Healthcare Improvement, June 2006, 1–3.

Glossary

Acuity: The level of severity of an illness or how sick a person is

Admission: A term for staying in the hospital when the patient is too sick to return home.

Ancillary: Departments within a healthcare system that provide necessary support to the patient care process. Examples include Radiology, Physical Therapy and Lab services

Aortic Dissection: A serious, but uncommon condition where the aorta tears due to weakness in the aortic wall. Chronic high blood pressure can cause this weakness. If the dissection is caught early enough, it can be treated with medications to lower blood pressure and prevent further weakening or surgery to reconstruct the aorta.

Appendicitis: A blockage in the lining of the appendix usually leads to infection that causes sudden pain in the lower abdomen. Treatment is typically the removal of the appendix.

Arrhythmia: Abnormal heart rhythm that can have many causes. Treatment may or may not be required depending on the severity of the arrhythmia but can include medication, implantable devices or the use of electrical impulses.

Artificial variability: The result of imposing poorly managed processes or systems on patient flow. Processes that are set up and unnecessarily constrained by hours of operation, schedules of certain individuals, work methods that create batching and the way emergencies are dealt with.

Atrial fibrillation: A very common condition where the heartbeat is irregular and results in poor blood flow. Symptoms are typically chest pain or shortness of breath. Treatment can include medications or minimally invasive surgery to adjust the heart rhythms.

Bariatric: Relating to the treatment of obesity

Baseline: Refers to the initial data, or what improvements are compared against

Bed-czar (or Central Bed Manager): The individual or department that directs bed placement throughout the facility. Most, if not all bed requests are reviewed and determined on a patient by patient basis and managed to be executed in a timely fashion.

Bi-Pap: Bi-level positive airway pressure is a machine used to support airway pressure (and assist in breathing)

Bottlenecks: The point in a process where everything slows down. That particular point cannot keep up with the demand, and can result in congestion and longer processing times

Boarder: A patient staying in a non-traditional area for the type of care they are receiving due to capacity restraints in the health care facility. A patient waiting for a bed on an Inpatient unit may board in the Emergency Department until a room becomes available, or a patient coming out of surgery may board in the recovery area until a surgical bed is ready.

Case Manager: Individual responsible for facilitating the collaboration between the patient, family, and resources, ensuring that their health needs are met in a thorough and cost effective way.

Catheterization Laboratory (Cath Lab): an examination room in a hospital or clinic with diagnostic imaging equipment used to visualize the arteries of the heart and the chambers of the heart and treat any stenosis or abnormality found.

Cholecystitis: Inflammation of the gallbladder that is often caused by gallstones and can be treated by removal of the gallbladder.

Chronic Obstructive Pulmonary Disease (COPD): A very common group of diseases that affect the lungs and make it difficult to breathe.

Complex care patients: Patients requiring more than a standard discharge home or to another facility. Can be due to financial complications, social issues or convoluted medical needs.

Compliance: Department of a hospital responsible for monitoring the operations of the facility and ensuring that all regulations are met. Also report out to several government and licensing agencies on a regular basis

Co-morbid condition: One or more conditions that exist simultaneously with the patient's primary condition

Core measures: A set of metrics determined by CMS that track the standards of care that are scientifically researched, and evidence based. Measures are submitted quarterly to CMS and then publicly reported to aid in transparency and stimulate improvement efforts.

Commercial Insurers: Also referred to as private insurance. It is insurance that is NOT paid for by the Federal Government

Consults: A visit to the patient usually done by a specialist in order to provide a review or recommendation on a specific element of their diagnosis.

Congestive Heart Failure (CHF): A very common condition where the heart stops pumping blood as well as it should. Heart failure can be caused by disease or infection or the instance of a heart attack. Treatment ranges from management of lifestyle and medications to bypass surgery or a heart transplant.

Coronary Artery Bypass Graft (CABG): A procedure used to treat blockages due to Coronary Artery Disease where pieces of other veins are used to reroute blood around the artery.

Demand level staffing: Developing a staffing plan that considers the demand (# of patients per hour typically) and assigns the calculated number of FTEs required.

Diagnosis Related Group (DRG): A classification system that assigns a certain cost to specific illnesses and their treatments which a hospital is then billed for

Direct Admission: A patient that is directly sent by their Primary Care Physician to be admitted to the hospital.

Disposition: The determination made by a patient care teams of where they will be placed. A disposition can be in regard to the level of care a patient needs in the hospital (ICU, observation service, Inpatient unit), or the level of care required upon discharge (ex. skilled nursing facility, rehab)

Elective procedure: A non-emergent surgical procedure that is scheduled in advance

Environmental services: Hospital department responsible for laundry, disposal and general housekeeping

EP Study: Electrophysiology study is used to test the heart for arrhythmia Electrocardiogram (EKG)**:** A non-invasive procedure where electrodes are placed all over the body to measure electrical activity all over the heart. The results are used to diagnose various heart conditions

Flex space: An area in the hospital where care is not traditionally given but can be used temporarily during times of high census. Can refer to patient beds in the hallways, or in other alcoves appropriate for care delivery.

HbA1C: Refers to glycated hemoglobin and is used to determine what a patient's blood sugar levels have been over time

Hemodialysis: A treatment for kidney failure where the blood is mechanically cycled through membrane to remove wastes and extra fluid.

High risk: Can be defined by a range of criteria, usually agreed upon conditions specific to the scenario. Often includes elderly, history of disease, co morbidities, and social issues.

History and physical: The initial evaluation of a patient where information is gathered regarding their current condition and a physical examination is performed

Hospitalists: Physicians who provide the general medical care of hospitalized patients

Home care: Services provided by an outside organization designed to support the patient in transitioning back into their home environment after a hospital stay. Home care can include activities such as wound care, rehabilitation, or pain management

Huddle: A brief, usually stand up meeting that can be used to review daily activities, goals, and identify barriers for a process.

Hyper emesis: A complication of pregnancy affecting less than 5% of women. Symptoms are severe nausea, vomiting and dehydration. Treatment is often an IV for hydration and nutrition.

Hypotension: Abnormal low blood pressure. Several causes such as heart problems, dehydration or severe infection. Typically, the underlying issue is treated, not the low blood pressure.

Hypoxia: A condition where the entire body or just one region is deprived of oxygen.

ICU: Intensive Care Unit-treats patients requiring a higher level of care within a hospital

InterQual Criteria: A Medicare tool used to determine if a hospital admission is medically necessary. The criteria consider the severity of the illness and complexity of the treatment to decide if a hospital stay was truly required for the patient.

Isolation: Precautions taken for patients with infectious or contagious diseases

Left Without Treatment (LWOT): A patient that leaves the healthcare facility before being treated.

Leveling: the process of looking at the surgical schedule of a facility and based on patient length of stay and procedure length, optimizing the number and type of surgeries each day to maximize capacity.

Medicaid: A state run insurance program for qualifying low-income individuals. Can vary state to state.

Medicare: Health insurance that is provided by the Federal Government for people 65 and older.

Medication Administration Record (MAR): A document in the patient's medical record stating all of the medications that have been given to the patient in a healthcare facility

Medication reconciliation: A process where the patient's medication orders are compared to the medications, they are actually taking

MRSA: a contagious and antibiotic-resistant staph bacterium that leads to potentially dangerous infection Methicillin Resistant Staphylococcus Auerus (WebMD)

Natural variability: Due to the time of day, differences in symptoms that patients present with, the pace at which individuals work, institutions seek to manage natural variability as there is no way to eliminate it.

Nursing Assessment: The collection and analysis of information on a patient's physical, social, and psychological condition

OR: Operating Room

Pacers: Term for a pacemaker. A device placed in the chest used to regulate the hearts contractions

Palliative care: Designed to provide the most comfortable care to the patient and family in the final stages of life. Often includes medication management, transfer to peaceful surroundings, and limited interventions.

Patient Protection and Affordable Care Act (PPACA): Statute signed into law in March 2010 with the goals of providing more affordable coverage to a greater number of Americans, improving the quality of health care and health insurance, regulating the health insurance industry, and reducing health care spending in the US

Pharmacokinetics: Refers to how the body responds and processes a drug

Pneumothorax: The rare condition of a collapsed lung that can be caused by a chest injury, medical procedures or lung disease. Treatment is to relieve the pressure on the lungs which in some cases can happen on its own. Other times it may include surgery to remove the excess air.

Post Anesthesia Care Unit (PACU): A unit usually near the operating rooms, designed to care for patients as they recover from anesthesia

Post-Acute Myocardial Infarction: Commonly referred to as a heart attack-occurs when blood stops pumping to a certain area of the heart causing damage. Myocardial Infarctions can be caused by smoking, a sedentary lifestyle, other disease as well as genetics. The treatments depend on the extent of the blockage and can range from

Pressers: Medication that increases blood pressure

Private Internists: A physician practicing medicine that is employed independent of a hospital

Pulmonary Embolus: The blockage of an artery in the lungs by a blood clot. Can be caused by lack of movement, cancer or surgical procedures. Drugs or procedures can be used to break up the clot and measures can be taken to prevent blood clots from forming.

Pyelonephritis: A kidney infection that results when a UTI progresses upwards in the urinary tract. Most cases can be treated with antibiotics.

Queue: A line up of people waiting for their turn

Rehab centers: Facility for patients that require additional recovery prior to returning to their homes following a hospital stay and/or surgical procedure. Recovery Audit Contractor (RAC): A Medicare program set up to review payments made under the Fee for Service plans and identify those that may be inappropriate

Reimbursement: Payment that the hospital or healthcare provider receives from the covering insurance provider or government payer, for care given during a patient's visit

Scatter bed Model: A way of providing care for observation level of care patients. Instead of grouping these patients together, scatter bed refers to the patients being placed all throughout the hospital, with no designated area for observation patients.

Semi-private room: A room shared by two patients

Standard work: Documentation that outlines the step by step process to be followed in order to obtain a certain result

Subspecialty: A specific field within a specialty. Commonly seen in Internal Medicine, Cardiology and Neurology.

Surge: The state of a hospital that is functioning at or above its typical capacity levels. This situation requires heightened attention from all disciplines in order to continue providing good care to its patient population. Additional resources may be required to provide the necessary care in times of high patient census

STEMI: ST Segment Elevation Myocardial Infarction is the more serious type of heart attack. Characterized by an elevated ST segment on an echocardiogram which indicates a large piece of heart muscle is being damaged

Telemetry: Automatic monitoring

Transfer: Refers to a patient that requires a higher level, or different care than their current location is capable of, is transferred to another location

Urinary Tract Infection (UTI): A condition common to females where an infection develops in the kidneys, ureter, bladder or urethra. Treatment is typically antibiotics.

VRE: Vancomycin-resistant enterococci (VRE) are a type of bacteria called enterococci that have developed resistance to many antibiotics, especially vancomycin.

Index

Note: Page numbers in *italic* indicate figures.

H

I

J

L

M

N

O

T

U

V

W

For Product Safety Concerns and Information please contact our EU
representative GPSR@taylorandfrancis.com
Taylor & Francis Verlag GmbH, Kaufingerstraße 24, 80331 München, Germany

www.ingramcontent.com/pod-product-compliance
Ingram Content Group UK Ltd.
Pitfield, Milton Keynes, MK11 3LW, UK
UKHW022203190926
475702UK00003B/180
* 9 7 8 0 3 6 7 7 0 8 6 0 3 *